Society, Medicine and Religion in the *Sacred Tales* of Aelius Aristides

Mnemosyne

Supplements

Monographs on Greek and Latin Language and Literature

VOLUME 341

The titles published in this series are listed at brill.nl/mns

Society, Medicine and Religion in the *Sacred Tales* of Aelius Aristides

By

Ido Israelowich

BRILL

LEIDEN · BOSTON
2012

Library of Congress Cataloging-in-Publication Data

Israelowich, Ido, 1972-
Society, medicine and religion in the sacred tales of Aelius Aristides / by Ido Israelowich.
pages cm. – (Mnemosyne supplements ; volume 341)
Includes bibliographical references and index.
ISBN 978-90-04-22908-2 (hardback : alkaline paper) – ISBN 978-90-04-22944-0 (e-book)
1. Aristides, Aelius. Sacred teachings. 2. Medicine, Greek and Roman–History. I. Title. II. Series: Mnemosyne, bibliotheca classica Batava. Supplementum ; v. 341.

PA3874.A7Z5 2012
885'.01–dc23

2012006305

This publication has been typeset in the multilingual "Brill" typeface. With over 5,100 characters covering Latin, IPA, Greek, and Cyrillic, this typeface is especially suitable for use in the humanities. For more information, please see www.brill.nl/brill-typeface.

ISSN 0169-8958
ISBN 978 90 04 22908 2 (hardback)
ISBN 978 90 04 22944 0 (e-book)

This book is printed on acid-free paper.

In memory of my grandfather,
Isaac Israelowich

CONTENTS

ACKNOWLEDGEMENTS

This study of society, medicine and religion in the *Sacred Tales* of Aelius Aristides began as an Oxford doctoral thesis. My initial intention was to examine the work of Aristides in the context of the Second Sophistic, but, in the course of the work, it became clear that the *Sacred Tales*' medical context must take precedence. In turn, the nature of Aristides' experiences while being ill raised the question of the relations between medicine and religion in the world of Aelius Aristides. My doctoral supervisors, Alan Bowman and Ewen Bowie, offered their help and advice throughout this intellectual process and I am very grateful to them for their assistance. The comments of my examiners, Simon Price and Michael Trapp, then proved invaluable in the process of turning my thesis into this monograph. Both the Faculty of Classics at Oxford and the Department of Classics in Tel Aviv University have provided me with stimulating and encouraging environments in which to write and research, and I would like to say special thanks to the libraries at both institutions. I would also like to acknowledge the financial assistance I received from the AVI Foundation, Anglo-Israel Association, St Cross College and Wadham College. Finally I want to thank my colleagues, friends and family, and partner Angela Davis for their patience and support.

INTRODUCTION

This study examines the themes of society, medicine and religion in the work of Aelius Aristides, with particular reference to his *Sacred Tales*. It investigates how Aristides envisaged his medical condition and the terms he used to comprehend and describe it. It also questions how, according to the *Sacred Tales*, medical knowledge and medical practice were conceived of in the Graeco-Roman world and whom society recognised as authoritative in offering health-care. Beyond this it also considers the relations between medicine and religion as depicted in the *Sacred Tales* and asks whether the *Sacred Tales* indicate a dichotomy between religion and medicine. Finally, it assesses the relationship between Aristides' experience of being ill and his religious experience.

Aristides was born in Mysia in Asia Minor, in the year Hadrian succeeded Trajan, and into a family of wealth and local political power. He gained the best possible education, excelled in his studies and aspired to the fame and glory a career as a rhetor could offer.[1] His promising career was brought to an unfortunate halt, however, due to severe illness when Aristides was only twenty-six years of age. He then spent the next few years convalescing in the Pergamene Asclepieion, having been invited to the temple by the god himself after physicians both in Rome and Smyrna failed to provide him with an effective treatment, an accurate prognosis or conclusive diagnosis.[2] While at the temple Aristides resumed scholarly activity,[3] but he never fully regained his health. According to the *Sacred Tales*, the special relationship between Asclepius and Aristides was cemented during the first revelation in the winter of 144 CE, and Aristides consulted the god on various issues from then onwards.

Aristides believed himself to be ill for the better part of his adult life. Many of the experiences he recorded in the *Sacred Tales* revolved around his medical condition and the measures he took to improve it. The medical

---

1 For the biography of Aristides see Behr (1994). For the composition of the *Sacred Tales* Behr (1968) is paramount. Puech (2002) 138–145 has collected all the epigraphical evidence relevant to Aristides. For more general background concerning the role of the Greek sophists in the Roman Empire see Bowersock (1969) with Bowie (1982) and Brunt (1994).

2 Aristid. *Or.* 48.5–7 K. *C.* December 144 CE.

3 Aristid. *Or.* 50.17–30 K.

context is therefore no less relevant when considering the work of Aristides than the social, linguistic and literary milieu of the Second Sophistic or a history of the Roman Empire under the Antonines. The works of ancient physicians, from the Hippocratic authors to Galen, as well as other corroborating evidence from Graeco-Roman medicine, will therefore be used as a point of reference for evaluating the testimony of Aristides. Particular attention will be paid to the manner in which Aristides understood his medical condition, the choices he made concerning his medical treatments, and his identification of those authoritative enough to assist him.

Another framework in which the *Sacred Tales* belong is that of Graeco-Roman religion. Aristides was a devout worshipper of Asclepius and his comprehension of his medical condition was intrinsically connected to his religious beliefs. The *Sacred Tales* contain many descriptions of daily life in the Pergamene Asclepieion, of the range of medical and religious services provided in the temple and elsewhere, and of its cultic habits. The role of dreams in divination is also significant. Aristides understood divination in general, and divination through dreams in particular, as being an obvious truth. Therefore an evaluation of the evidential force of his work is incomplete without placing Aristides in this context as well.

The broader implications of the issues to be raised here concern Graeco-Roman medicine during the high empire and the conceptual scheme in which medicine operated. Also relevant is the particular nature of the dialogue between medicine and religion at this time. Finally, a study of society, medicine and religion in Aristides' *Sacred Tales* will cast light on a number of more general issues concerning culture and society in the latter half of the second century CE. For example, it will contribute to our understanding of the religious climate under the Antonines, the level of popularity of the cult of Asclepius and the implications of this appeal. The *Sacred Tales* also provide valuable information concerning the great plague of 165 CE and its impact on the province of Asia through Aristides' personal testimony about its devastating effects on himself and his household in his Mysian estate. Aristides' position on all these matters will therefore be considered and contextualised. It will then be possible to assess the contribution Aristides' *Sacred Tales* can make to historical research on medicine and religion.

The means available for and relevant to this work begin, naturally, with an analysis of the *Sacred Tales* themselves. In these *Tales* Aristides portrayed, in a highly personal manner and in great detail, his ailments and the measures he undertook to overcome them. Encounters with a wide range of health-care providers (physicians and priests, gymnastic trainers and experts in the interpretation of dreams), alongside the treatments they prescribed and the outcomes of these therapeutic measures, are elaborately depicted and offer a vivid testimony of being ill and seeking medical help, unparalleled among the evidence to have reached us from classical antiquity. With the help of a wide range of corroborating evidence, such as the works of ancient physicians, the votive inscriptions from the temples of Asclepius and from other centres of temple-healing and many other kinds of testimonies, I will attempt to contextualise the *Sacred Tales* and determine how representative a picture they offer of the practice of medicine in the world of Aelius Aristides.

In addition, this study of the historical value of the *Sacred Tales* also builds upon other areas of scholarly activity. Some of the key themes of this study, such as the relationship between society and culture, the meaning of religion and mythology and their role in society, and the function of language as a medium of representation, have also received the attention of researchers outside the field of classical studies. Sociology and anthropology provide students of Graeco-Roman culture in general, and of Aelius Aristides in particular, with powerful tools of analysis.[4] The study of culture and religion by the anthropologist Clifford Geertz and Arthur Kleinman's analysis of *Patients and Healers in the Context of Culture* will be of use, especially when looking into the description of Aristides' malady in the *Sacred Tales*.[5] Likewise applicable to the study of the religious experience of Aristides, particularly when coming to appreciate the influences of Graeco-Roman society and culture, are some of the analytical tools that philosophy of language and sociology can provide. The ground-breaking works of Ludwig Wittgenstein and Maurice Halbwachs demonstrate the seminal role of society in shaping the mental world of individuals and the impossibility of private language and, by implication, private religion.[6] Such conclusions have significant implications for a study of Aristides.

This study's principal methodology is a critical analysis of the *Sacred Tales* themselves. Some modern scholars, following a few hostile scholia

[4] For the heuristic contribution of anthropology to the ancient historian see Momigliano (1966) 581.

[5] For the course of anthropological approaches to the study of religion see especially Baal (1971); Banton (1966); Evans-Pritchard (1965); Firth (1973); La Barre (1972); Skorupski (1976); Wallase (1966) and Poole (1986). Attention should also be paid to the works of Mary Douglas, James Fernandez, Clifford Geertz, Claude Lévi-Strauss, Melford E. Spiro and Victor W. Turner. Finally, some aspects of the dialogue between the approaches of anthropology towards religion and that of other disciplines are discussed by Bianki (1973), Spiro (1973) and in the works of Jonathan Z. Smith.

[6] Wittgenstein (1968); Halbwachs (1992).

to the *Sacred Tales* envisage a 'vain and neurotic' Aristides.[7] Other scholars choose to emphasise the religious experience of Aristides as genuine.[8] An analysis of the reasons for the *Sacred Tales* composition and an understanding of the work's elusive subject matter are therefore essential to this study. Being the work of an orator who publicly delivered many of his speeches, it is crucial to ask how much of what Aristides said can be taken as his genuine views and beliefs, and how much should be seen as an orator anticipating what his audience wanted to hear. In other words, does the work of Aristides reveal his own views or those of his audience?

In consequence, it is necessary initially to enquire into the role of the *Sacred Tales* in Aristides' corpus. Were they meant to be published? Who was Aristides' audience? Aristides himself is not clear about these issues. A comment in which Aristides advises all his readers who were unfortunate enough to suffer similar illnesses to his own to look for the actual prescriptions Asclepius sent him in his notebooks, raises more questions than it answers.[9] Did these notebooks really exist, and, if so, did Aristides see them as medical writings? Just before this cryptic advice, Aristides announced the aim of this work, namely to tell of all the benefactions Asclepius bestowed upon him.[10] Is this, therefore, a work of eulogy to a benevolent god, or could Aristides have had a hidden agenda? After all, Aristides was a rhetor arguing that Asclepius himself ordered him to resume the practice of writing and declaiming.[11] Moreover, while in the Pergamene Asclepieion the god is said to have actively trained the ailing Aristides,[12] who, in turn, chose to entitle his period in the temple his *cathedra*.[13] It is a highly unusual way of describing a time of convalescence and a term with connotations of the professional practice of rhetoric.[14] Could it be that Aristides tried to promote himself as a rhetor by arguing that Asclepius was his teacher and patron? It is hoped that the remarks of ancient readers of the *Sacred Tales*, such as Philostratus and Libanius, Sopater and Synesius, may provide some answers to these questions.

---

[7] Weiss (1998) 10. See also Behr (1968) 115; Schmid (1887–1897) vol. ii, pp. 10–11; Weinreich (1914) 601. For the scholia see Dindorf (1829) 343–344.

[8] Festugière (1954) 97–98; Dodds (1965) 43–45; Perkins (1995) 175, 183.

[9] Aristid. *Or*. 48.3 K.

[10] Aristid. *Or*. 48.1–4 K.

[11] Aristid. *Or*. 50.17–30 K; Bompaire (1989) 36–39 collects the passages in which Asclepius functions as Aristides' 'maître de rhétorique'.

[12] Ibid.

[13] Aristid. *Or*. 48.70, 49.44 K.

[14] See pp. 109–111.

Recent historical analyses can likewise provide assistance in the endeavour of deciphering Aristide's intentions. Alexia Petsalis-Diomidis' innovative study of the *Sacred Tales* argues convincingly that the text should be read within the context of the Second Sophistic and that Aelius Aristides was anything but an eccentric author.[15] The following study and that of Petsalis-Diomidis differ in the strategies they adopt to demonstrate this point, however. While addressing the medical discourses and the religious framework of the Asclepian cult, Petsalis-Diomidis's main focus is on the themes of the body and travel, employing a broad range of literary texts and archaeological evidence from the Pergamene Asclepieion in support. In contrast this book deals specifically with medicine and health care and their relationship to religion, situating the *Sacred Tales* within the Graeco-Roman medical cannon. Taken together, these complementary approaches offer a more comprehensive analysis of the *Sacred Tales* and their context.

Modern scholarship on Graeco-Roman medicine also offers valuable insights when contextualizing the medical aspects of the *Sacred Tales*. The two volumes of collected essays edited by Philip van der Eijk, Manfred Horstmanshoff and Piet Schrijvers, on ancient medicine in its socio-cultural context contain a wide range of studies of the social, institutional and geographical aspects of medical practice in classical antiquity, about the religious and magical attitudes towards disease and healing, about medicine as a science and its relation to philosophy, and, finally, about the linguistic and literary attributes of classical medical writings.[16] As such, the collection provides an essential background to this study of Aristides. Likewise a collection of essays by Mirko Grmek[17] includes many significant contributions to the understanding of the conceptualisation of pathological events and about various other areas of ancient medicine.[18] Évelyne Samama's book about the physician in the Greek world, which incorporates a large collection of relevant inscriptions, sheds light on some of the social characteristics of Aristides' interactions with his physicians, as do the earlier

[15] My debt to the study of Petsalis-Diomidis (2010) is demonstrated by the references to her work throughout. Though Petsalis-Diomidis focused on the themes of travel and landscape, while the present study focuses on medicine and health care there is, I think, an added value in reading these two studies together.

[16] Van der Eijk, Horstmanshoff & Scrijvers (1995).

[17] Originally published in French in 1983 and translated into English in 1989.

[18] Grmek (1989).

works of Ludwig Edelstein.[19] More general studies of medicine in classical antiquity such as Giuseppe Penso's study of medicine in the Roman world; Antje Krug's archaeologically-oriented study of ancient medicine; and Vivian Nutton's comprehensive book on ancient medicine also provides essential context.[20] Finally, an article by Jacques Jouanna on the interpretation of dreams and the theory of micro-macro cosmos in the Hippocratic treatise *On Regimen* provides a good starting point for tracing the interrelation between medicine and other disciplines, notably divination, particularly when it comes to medical applications of dream-interpretation in classical antiquity.[21] This book will build upon this existing scholarship, but will also extend existing knowledge through a detailed of the medical aspects of Aristides' *Sacred Tales*.

According to the *Sacred Tales*, Aristides viewed his dreams as divine messages from the god of medicine, Asclepius, and utilised the information they contained to regain his lost health. Furthermore, if we are to believe the testimony of Aristides, he enjoyed the support of various health-care providers (such as physicians and priests) and institutions (such as the Asclepieion itself) in so doing. Here too modern scholarship proves beneficial when contextualizing Aristides' views and for evaluating the merit of the *Sacred Tales* as evidence for the relation between medicine and divination in Aristides' world. More than a century ago Auguste Bouché-Leclercq published his monumental and still relevant work on divination in classical antiquity, which includes detailed discussions of the practice of divination through dreams, the inducement of the gods to send dreams by incubation and the medical application of these rites.[22] In 1900 Ludwig Deubner published a study concerning the habit of incubation, which demonstrated that it was widely practised among pagans, and among Christians, all through classical antiquity and well into the early Middle Ages.[23] More than half a century later Eric Dodds looked into the ancient interpretation of dreams as divine messages in his works on the Greeks' attitudes towards the irrational, and on some aspects of pagan and Christian religion during the second and third centuries.[24] Antonius Kessels' meticulous study of the ancient systems of

---

[19] Samama (2003); Edelstein (1967) includes some important studies of the author on various aspects of ancient medicine.

[20] Penso (1984); Krug (1985); Nutton (2004).

[21] Jouanna (1998).

[22] Bouché-Leclercq (1879).

[23] Deubner (1900).

[24] Dodds (1951) (1965).

dream-classification demonstrated that ancient philosophers and doxographers were intrigued by the dream-phenomenon and that although not all ancient treatises about dreams shared the same taxonomy and identical views as to the sub-categories of dreams, they all accepted an essential division of dreams into mantic and non-mantic. Kessels was also able to demonstrate that ancient physicians, who were equally interested in the nature of dreams, shared the vocabulary and taxonomy of the philosophers and doxographers when looking into the nature of dreams. Indeed, distinguished medical authorities such as Hippocrates, Herophilus and Galen accepted the division of dreams into mantic and non-mantic and recognised the importance of the latter category to the physician's work.[25] Simon Price surveyed the differences between ancient and modern approaches to dreams, focusing on the classical approaches and their relevance to our understanding of Graeco-Roman religions and medicine.[26] Patricia Cox Miller has examined the ways in which dreams conveyed meaning in late antiquity and the ancient hermeneutics of dreaming.[27] William Harris has inquired into the Roman opinions about the truthfulness of dreams, and Gil Renberg has looked into the language of the votive inscriptions which were incited by dreams.[28] All of these works and many others will be utilised in the following chapters.

One additional branch of scholarship which will be used throughout this monograph concerns the religions of classical antiquity. Aristides was of Greek origin and a Roman citizen who wrote and published a number of epideictic speeches and prose hymns to many of the deities of the Greek pantheon. He was also a devout worshipper of Asclepius. Most of the experiences he described in the *Sacred Tales* also had religious meaning. Therefore in reading this work I will make constant reference to and use of relevant modern scholarship, such as Ludwig and Emma Edelstein's study of Asclepius, Price's book on Greek religion and the study of Mary Beard, John North and Price on the religions of the Roman world in order to contextualise the experiences of Aristides and to measure their ability to represent either typical or eccentric religious behaviour.[29] For more specific issues, such as whether Aristides' devotion to Asclepius qualifies as conversion, the

---

25 Kessels (1969) 424 and *passim*.
26 Price (2004).
27 Cox Miller (1994).
28 Harris (2003); Renberg (2003).
29 L. & E. Edelstein (1945); Price (1999); Beard, North & Price (1998).

representation of religious themes in Graeco-Roman art, the popularity of the cult of Asclepius and many others, modern scholarship offers many valuable contributions as I allude to throughout.

In the first chapter I look into the *Sacred Tales* as a text, asking when, how and why they were written and what their textual characteristics can reveal. I ask whether Aristides followed any pre-existing literary patterns when writing the *Sacred Tales* and, if so, whether these literary choices disclose something of their author's intentions. I examine whether the Graeco-Roman literary tradition dictated any of Aristides' descriptions and choices of themes when composing the texts. In addition I question whether these influences were restricted to matters of form or whether their traces can be found in the province of content as well. In order to accomplish this aim I locate the *Sacred Tales* in the Graeco-Roman literary tradition. This preliminary textual analysis is crucial for the following chapters of this study. Two general questions that are posed throughout the work concern, firstly, Aristides' intentions when writing the *Sacred Tales*, and, secondly, how representative the *Sacred Tales* were, both in their form and content, of their time.

The next chapter addresses the themes of society, disease and medicine in the *Sacred Tales*. In the *Sacred Tales* Aristides writes of how he was ill for the majority of his adult life. He also describes his encounters with a range of health-care providers including physicians, priests, gymnastic trainers and the gods themselves. This chapter therefore retraces the grid of knowledge which directed Aristides' understanding of his medical condition and guided his search for remedies. It asks whether Aristdes' comprehension of his illness, his appeals to the healers he thought were most suitable to offer him treatment, and the actual treatments he underwent were common to his day and age. I begin by offering a theoretical framework for such a study and discuss its heuristic capacities, but also its shortcomings. I then proceed towards a general outline of Graeco-Roman medicine, which provides the context for the analysis of the *Tales*. According to the *Sacred Tales*, many of Aristides' treatments were prescribed to him by Asclepius through dreams. Furthermore, in the *Sacred Tales* Aristides reports that the health-care providers he consulted encouraged him to accept these divine remedies and were well-disposed towards the use of dreams in medical treatment. In consequence it is necessary to read the text in the context of prevailing views about the nature of dreams in classical antiquity, their use in medical practice and their role in divination. This general review will therefore follow the discussion of Graeco-Roman medicine. I then move on to consider the *Sacred Tales* themselves, asking how the sick, medicine and physicians are conceived of within them. Finally, I endeavour to compose a medical biography of Aristides.

The third chapter examines the religious modes of Aristides' experiences as they are depicted in the *Sacred Tales*. It asks whether his behaviour was a result of religious extremism and if his cultic habits fell under the category of 'private' or 'personal' religion. Referring to the study of religion as a cultural system Geertz has noted that, 'the notion that religion tunes human actions to an envisaged cosmic order and projects images of cosmic order onto the plane of human experience is hardly novel'. 'But', Geertz continues, 'it is hardly investigated either, so that we have very little idea of how, in empirical terms, this particular miracle is accomplished'.[30] Most if not all of the therapeutic measures Aristides undertook were described by him as being religiously motivated. This third chapter therefore provides an overall analysis of religion in the *Sacred Tales* and functions as commentary on the second chapter. These latter two chapters, alongside the first chapter on the text itself, aim to achieve a better understanding of the interrelation between medicine, religion and society in the world of the *Sacred Tales*.

---

[30] Geertz (1973) 90.

CHAPTER ONE

AELIUS ARISTIDES AND THE *SACRED TALES*

Introduction

Aelius Aristides composed the *Sacred Tales* in the early 170s, during the sixth decade of his life, and despite their unusual contents, the *Sacred Tales* are, in many ways, a work representative of an educated member of the Greek upper class in the province of Asia in the second half of the second century CE. The *Sacred Tales* have been read by modern scholars as reflecting some general trends of religious change that occurred during this time.[1] Half a century ago André-Jean Festugière recognised in Aristides' *Tales* evidence for the widespread existence of private religions among the Greeks and a decade later Eric Dodds used the testimony of the *Sacred Tales* to describe the latter years of the reign of Marcus Aurelius as an age of anxiety.[2] More recent scholars, such as Wolf Liebeschuetz, have tended to accept the verdict of Festugière and Dodds, at least when it comes to the ability of Aristides' work to mirror the religious climate of his age.[3] The *Sacred Tales* can

---

[1] For a history of pagan religion during this period see Lane Fox (1986) 64–101; Beard, North & Price vol. i (1998) 211–312; Liebeschuetz (2000).

[2] Festugière (1954) 85–104; Dodds (1965) 41–45 and *passim*. Similar views to Dodds' can be seen in his contemporary Phillips, who professed that the *Sacred Tales* are 'unique in surviving literature as a [record of] a nervous hypochondriac and lifelong devotee of Asclepius' Phillips (1952) 23; Lane Fox, loc. cit. is more critical of the use of the term 'anxiety' for describing this era. His preference is 'an age of anger'. The grounds for this disagreement are, however, mainly poetic and do not challenge the picture portrayed by Dodds.

[3] Liebeschuetz (2000) 1004; see also MacMullen (1976) 37. Aristides' belief (i) that divination is possible; (ii) that dreams often include messages from a deity and (iii) that the gods send remedies to their sick worshippers via dreams and other forms of divination was shared by none other than Marcus Aurelius himself. The emperor himself actually received a remedy from the gods by a dream, as we learn from his own testimony: 'that by the agency of dream I was given antidotes both of other kinds and against the spitting of blood and vertigo' (τὸ δι' ὀνειράτων βοηθήματα δοθῆναι ἄλλα τε καὶ ὡς μὴ πτύειν αἷμα καὶ μὴ ἰλιγγιᾶν) M.Ant. *Med.* 1.17.9. Similar views to those of Marcus are found in the letters of the emperor's friend and former tutor, Fronto, who wrote to the future emperor in 143–144 CE that the gods 'give their aid and show their power in dreams or mysteries, or healing, or oracles' (Fronto, *Ep.* 3.9 Naber, p. 47). Both these examples demonstrate that the belief in divination was widespread during Aristides' lifetime and that the connection between dreams and medicine, and between medicine and religion, was held to be valid by the most respectable people.

also be seen as representative of their times on other grounds. Their pure Attic dialect reflects a general inclination amongst Greek authors during the high empire, generally known as Atticism. The overall understanding of how dreams work and their use in the practice of divination, much like Aristides' religious habits and beliefs, were also typical of their age.[4] In addition, Aristides' focus on the body, which was analysed by Judith Perkins, Brooke Holmes, and Alexia Petsalis-Diomidis has been shown to be representative of this period.[5] In the following chapter I will assess the contribution the *Sacred Tales* can make to the history of medicine, religion and the interconnection between the two in the Graeco-Roman world.

Before one can proceed with such a study of society, medicine and religion in the *Sacred Tales*, some questions concerning the text itself must first be raised. In addition to the work's content, the form of the *Sacred Tales* is also pertinent. Aristides' choice of genre, his preference for a first-person narrative and his use of highly personal source materials such as his own medical history and dreams all have a distinct effect upon the reader which has to be acknowledged and addressed. Holmes' study of Aristides illegible body has demonstrated that one cannot take Aristides' narrative in the *Sacred Tales* at face value for tracing the author's medical history and that the theme of suffering, particularly when compared with that of Odysseus was consciously employed by a highly skilled author for self promotion.[6] Likewise, Aristides' avoidance of a systematically chronological narrative and the alternation between past and present events eliminates any sense of tension or suspense.[7] The reader of the *Sacred Tales* is told at the beginning of both the first and second *Tales* that Aristides was saved by Asclepius. The only gaps which the narrative therefore has to fill are those of detail; it

[4] Language and Atticism: Swain (1996) 17–64. Aristides' renown for his pure Attic style in late antiquity and early Byzantine era explains why so many of his works survived; Swain (1996) 254; Schmid (1887–1897) ii 7 n. 14, 14; Boulanger (1923) 452–457. Dreams: Price (2004) is seminal. For the changes in religious climate see Liebeschuetz (2000) 1001–1008.

[5] Perkins (1995); Holmes (2008); Petsalis-Diomidis (2008), (2010).

[6] Holmes (2008) 81–84, and *passim*.

[7] For a stimulating and authoritative discussion of the effects of the various forms of narrative sequences, and their ability to create a sense of tension and suspense see Sternberg (1977). More general works about narrative and narratology which are relevant here are: Bakhtin (1981); Genette (1980); Ricoeur (1984); Bal (1984); White (1987) and Cohan and Shires (1988). Prince (1987) and Cuddon (1991) provide useful dictionaries to the terms of literary theory and narratology. De Jong and Sullivan (1994) discuss the use of literary theory in the field of classical studies. Hornblower (1994) exemplified the usefulness of modern theories of narratology to the study of Thucydides and a recent book by Schmitz (2006) summarizes the major schools of critical theory and is aimed specifically at classicists.

informs the reader as to how this salvation took place. This absence of tension and suspense, I shall argue, colours the *Sacred Tales* with an aretalogical character.

Further questions to be raised and addressed have to do with Aristides' prospective readership and the actual effect of the *Sacred Tales* upon its ancient readers. Unlike his record of the dreams themselves,[8] Aristides claimed that he wrote the *Sacred Tales* for publication.[9] This claim is not in itself unprecedented. Pearcy has pointed out that the combination of dream-narrative and praise of the god was not unusual when Aristides was writing, particularly in the context of the cults of Sarapis and Asclepius.[10] In fact, as Pearcy noted, one of the functionaries of the cult of Serapis was the *aretalogos*, who celebrated the god's miracles.[11] Indeed, by 177 CE, when Aristides delivered his speech *Address Regarding Asclepius*, he expected his audience to be familiar with his *Sacred Tales*.[12] Furthermore, Aristides must have been very proud of this work. He thought it worthy to ascribe the guidance and inspiration for its composition to no less an authority than Asclepius himself.[13] If one is to believe Aristides, he composed the *Sacred Tales* as a eulogy to Asclepius for providing him with a cure. In this chapter I will undertake a textual analysis of the *Sacred Tales*, inquiring about their date of composition and *raison d'être*. I will try to understand whether Aristides saw the *Sacred Tales* as a eulogy and nothing more, or whether he had an ulterior motive, such as commemorating himself as an orator by claiming Asclepius as his literary patron and, if so, what literary means he employed to this end. A critique of the text itself will form the core of this chapter, but considered in the context of votive offerings in centres of healing cults and the comments of the *Sacred Tales*' ancient readers. First I will assess the composition of the *Sacred Tales*. Secondly I will examine

---

8 Quet argued convincingly that Aristides did not intend to publish his dream-record (Quet [1993] 218–220) although Aristides himself exhorts his readers to consult these books: Aristid. *Or.* 48.8 K.

9 Aristid. Or. 48.8 K with Quet (1993) 226. However, the critique raised by Petsalis-Diomidis concerning the existence of the parchments and the record of the dreams themselves and dismissing it as a rhetorical sophistication of Aristides is not without reason; Petsalis-Diomidis (2010) 128. My argument here therefore concerns merely the intention of Aristides as an author and the imperssions he wished to create with his readers and not the objective and undisputable truth.

10 Pearcy (1988) 377.

11 Pearcy (1988) 377–378; *SIG* 1133 = I.*Delos* 2072.

12 Aristid. *Or.* 42.4 K.

13 Aristid. *Or.* 42.3 K. In the second *Sacred Tale* Arristides argued that the *Sacred Tales* enjoyed the seal of divine approval (ἐπισημαίνω s.v. *LSJ* IV. 3) *Or.* 48.9 K; Weiss (1998) 8.

the *Sacred Tales* as a work of autobiography. Thirdly I will address the readership of the *Tales*; and finally I will ask whether they can be best viewed as a narrative of redemption.

1. The Composition of the *Sacred Tales*

Date of Composition

Stephen Harrison argues that the *Sacred Tales* were certainly published after 170 CE.[14] Charles Behr dates them to 170–171 CE,[15] but Harrison, following Charles Weiss, considers 175–176 CE to be a more plausible date of publication.[16] As Harrison notes, the crucial piece of evidence is the identity of the Salvius mentioned at *Or*.48.9 K as τοῦ νῦν ὑπάτου 'the present consul'.[17] Behr's most recent reading of the passage[18] is: εἵς τῶν ὑπάτων, 'one of the consuls', and he interprets the reference as being to L. Salvius Julianus, the consul of 148 CE (*PIR* S 103).[19] In contrast, Weiss argues in favour of the transmitted text. He believes that Aristides' Salvius is the consul of 175 CE, P. Salvius Julianus (*PIR* S 104), possibly the son of the consul of 148 CE.[20] As Harrison notes, this would give a firm *terminus post quem* for the publication of *Sacred Tales* of 175 CE.[21] This mention of a presiding Roman consul in the *Sacred Tales* is hardly surprising. It must have helped Aristides to gain credibility for his story. Both the presence of such a distinguished and well-known figure in the Asclepieion, and the god's choice to reveal himself in his image were likely to have had a reassuring effect on both Aristides and Zosimus, as well as on the prospective readership of the *Sacred Tales*. It also provides

14 Harrison (2000) 3.

15 In both Behr (1968) and (1994).

16 Harrison (2000) 3. Weiss (1998) 37–46. In his thesis Weiss juxtaposes rather than compares the conversion narratives of Lucius and Aristides, and though he raises in his conclusion (163–165) the possibility that Apuleius knew Aristides (citing Harrison [1996]), he is equally happy to suggest that conversion is a generic experience of sophists, citing the cases of Isaeus (Philostr. *VS* 2.20) and Dio Chrysostom.

17 Harrison (2000) 3.

18 Behr has twice emended the passage.

19 See the discussion in Behr (1994) 1155–1163. His strongest argument is that the crucial reference occurs in a vision dated to 144 CE and that the consul of 175 CE would have then been a young boy, but such a thing would not be impossible, as Weiss (1998) 38 n. 55 argues.

20 Weiss (1998) 38–39; the date is also favoured by Bowersock (1969) 79–80 and by Avotins (1971) 348. ὕπατος is the regular Greek word for consul (cf. Mason [1974] 165–171). It is the only occurrence of this term in Aristides' work, excluding *Or*. 28.45; 47.30; 49.77 K where Aristides refers to Zeus.

21 Harrison (2000) 3.

modern scholars with significant help for the purposes of dating. According to Weiss, the *Sacred Tales* were intended to be presented to Marcus Aurelius and his son Commodus on their imperial tour of the eastern provinces of the Roman empire in 175–176 CE. During the tour, in spring 176 CE (cf. Philostratus *VS* 2.10), they met Aristides at Smyrna. Weiss asserts that the constant element of self-promotion in the work reflects, according to Weiss, Aristides' candidacy for the post of rhetorical tutor to the young Commodus.[22] Harrison concludes that this remains speculative, but a *terminus post quem* of 175 CE for the publication of the *Sacred Tales* seems not unlikely.[23]

Events from March 171 CE are the latest to have been included in the *Sacred Tales*.[24] The project of compiling the *Sacred Tales* itself was instigated by a dream Asclepius sent Aristides in the late 160s.[25] The first *Sacred Tale* appears to have been antecedent. The additional five soon followed.[26] It is possible that Aristides began with a more modest work in mind, maybe in the form of a eulogy to Asclepius, of the kind which was often found in the temples of the god.[27] The work expanded, however, and Aristides evidently embarked on a more ambitious plan, to describe as many events as he could in regard to Asclepius' assistance to improve his health. However, as Weiss suggested, the actual date of publication might have been a few years later than the last events recorded, if his reading of *Or.* 48.9 is accurate, and the Salvius Aristides referred to as a consul was P. Salvius Julianus. Neither Behr's suggested date of publication as 170–171 CE, nor Weiss' hypothesis is beyond dispute. However Aristides himself referred to the *Sacred Tales* in his encomium *Address Regarding Asclepius*,[28] which means that by the time the speech was delivered (January 177 CE) the *Sacred Tales* were already in circulation.

Method of Composition

Aristides kept a record of his dreams 'straight from the beginning' (εὐθὺς ἐξ ἀρχῆς),[29] as ordered by Asclepius when the god first revealed himself to him.[30] In fact, the actual documentation of god-sent dreams was not

---

22 Weiss (1998) 37–46.

23 Harrison (2000) 3.

24 Aristid. *Or.* 47.59; 49.34–36; 50.30; 50.68–69 K.

25 Aristid. *Or.* 48.2 K; Bompaire (1993) 199. Behr dated this dream to 166 CE, (1981–1986) ad loc.

26 Bompaire (1993) 199.

27 Cf. *IG* IV^2, 1. 121–122; Behr (1981–1986) vol. ii. p. 425.

28 Aristid. *Or.* 42.10 K.

29 Aristid. *Or.* 48.2 K.

30 Aristid. *Or.* 48.2–3; 49.26; 50.25, 39 K.

unique to Aristides. A letter of the physician Thessalus of Tralles to either Nero or Claudius records how common it was for taking writing materials into the incubation room for the sole purpose of recording dreams.[31] Two generations later, a papyrus written close to the time of Aristides has the Egyptian deity associated with Asclepius, Imoutheus, ordering one of his worshippers to write his praise for his divinity.[32] As demonstrated by Pearcy, P. *Oxy* 1381 bears some similarities with Aristides' *Sacred Tales*. Both its author and Aristides were urged to write by the god, and both narratives are a reworking of an earlier document.[33]

Aristides meticulously followed Asclepius' instruction to record his dreams, and even at times when he was unable to write himself, Aristides dictated the contents of his dreams as soon as they occurred.[34] Aristides did not intend his record of his dreams in the *Sacred Tales* to provide a medical history in which he described his symptoms and illnesses and how the dreams' contents affected them.[35] Indeed he confessed that his memories about some of the exact circumstances were obscure. Aristides did, however, claim to have kept a diary where he recorded his medical history and his reactions to his treatment, but this diary probably did not cover the entire time-span of the *Sacred Tales*. When composing the *Sacred Tales*, Aristides used this diary for information about the circumstances in which the dreams were delivered.[36] The record of the dreams themselves, however, was not available to Aristides at the time of writing the *Sacred Tales*, and, aside from the help his diary provided, he had to rely on his memory.[37] Aristides nonetheless can tell us that in its final form the record of the dreams included more than 300,000 lines 'but it is neither easy to go over them or to fit them into their proper chronology'.[38]

The ability of Aristides to recount his dreams, some of which dated back several decades, has caused some scholars to cast doubt on the authenticity and precision of Aristides' reporting. Behr (objecting to Wilamowitz and

---

[31] P. Boudreaux, *Catalogus Codicum Astrologum Graecorum*, 8.3, 132–153; Festugière (1967) 155–163.

[32] *P.* Oxy 1381.

[33] Pearcy (1988) 378; cf. Winkler (1985) 234–237.

[34] Aristid. *Or*. 48.2 K.

[35] Petsalis-Diomidis (2010) 122–124 has argued that the *Sacred Tales* have often been misunderstood due to what she referred to as 'over-realistic' readings.

[36] Diary: Aristid. *Or*. 47.4–57 K; Behr (1968) 116.

[37] Aristid. *Or*. 49.26 K.

[38] ἀλλ' οὔτ' ἐπελθεῖν δή που ῥᾴδιον αὐτὰς οὔτ' ἐφαρμόττειν ἑκάστοις ὅπως εἶχε τὰ τῶν χρόνων. Aristid. *Or*. 48.3 K.

supported by Björck), thought that Aristides had a strong memory, which enabled him to recall his dreams.[39] Pearcy called to mind the discrepancy between Aristides' record of his dreams (ἀπογραφή) which amounted to 300,000 lines and were not available to Aristides for the composition of the *Sacred Tales*, and his suggestion for the keen readers to consult his notebooks (διφθέρας). He concluded that the *apographai* and *diphtheras* did not refer to the same thing.[40] The *apographê* were seen by Pearcy and later by Holmes as the lost sourse of the *Sacred Tales* we now have, the record of the actual events.[41] 'The *apographê*', according to Pearcy, 'is a foil against which the existence of the narrative must be read. As a rejected way of telling the sotry, it increases the authority and persuasiveness of the narrative before us, and because this rejected way of telling was, as Aristides presents it, a voluminous transcription of reality, its rejection amounts to a rejection of the claims of reality on the narrative'.[42]

Quet also discusses the role of memory in the composition of the *Sacred Tales*,[43] as does Swain,[44] but none of the above scholars, when questioning Aristides' ability to recall old dreams, considered the unique difficulties of remembering dreams. Their doubts revolve solely around the power of memory itself, and do not address the hypothesis (which originated from Freudian psycho-analysis) that the mind imposes strong censorship on dream-remembrance.[45] Behr, however, rightly points out that the language of the dream-descriptions in the *Sacred Tales* is not typical of a Second Sophistic author, but more closely resembles a modern psychological text book.[46] One plausible explanation is, therefore, that Aristides recorded his dreams when they occurred and it is the memory of his written records, rather than that of his actual dreams, that the reader finds in the *Sacred Tales*.[47]

---

39 Behr (1968) 116; Wilamowitz-Möllendorf (1925) 344; Björck (1946) 307.

40 ἀπογραφή: 48. 3 K; διφθέρας: 48.8 K; Pearcy (1988) 380–381.

41 Pearcy (1988); Holmes (2008).

42 Pearcy (1988) 383.

43 Quet (1993) 220–226.

44 Swain (1996) 260–274.

45 Freud and his followers understood the dream to be a window to the unconscious. Forgetting a dream was therefore, taken to be a defence mechanism against unsettling notions.

46 This led Behr to assume that the dreams Aristides recorded were genuine and that Aristides actually remembered his dreams, because the language he uses to recall them is typical of a person recalling his dreams. Behr (1968) 117.

47 Remembering the records of his dreams, which Aristides meticulously put in writing each morning, solves the difficulty of overcoming the censorship the mind imposes. If to

Both Aristides' method of composition of the *Sacred Tales* and the thread of their narrative are hard to define. The *Sacred Tales* disorder events.[48] The order of the dream episodes in the text may not correspond to their chronological order or to their order in Aristides' notebooks.[49] The absence of a chronological sequence, the frequent digressions and the variety of topics covered in the *Sacred Tales* all indicate that Aristides did not attempt to write a history of his illness. He advised his readers who were interested in the prescriptions that Asclepius gave him for medical purposes to consult another of his works, stating:

> εἰ δέ τις τὰ ἀκριβέστατα γνῶναι βουλήσεται τῶν γεγενημένων ἡμῖν παρὰ τοῦ θεοῦ, ὥρα τὰς διφθέρας αὐτῷ ζητεῖν καὶ τὰ ὀνείρατα αὐτά. καὶ γὰρ ἰάματα παντὸς εἴδους καὶ διαλόγους τινὰς εὑρήσει καὶ λόγους ἐν μήκει καὶ φάσματα παντοῖα καὶ προρρήσεις ἁπάσας καὶ χρησμῳδίας περὶ παντοδαπῶν πραγμάτων, τὰς μὲν καταλογάδην, τὰς δὲ ἐν μέτροις γεγονυίας, καὶ χαρίτων πάντ' ἄξια τῷ θεῷ μειζόνων ἤ τις ἂν εἰκάσαι.[50]
>
> If someone will wish to know precisely what has befallen us from the god, it is time for him to seek out the parchment books and the dreams themselves. For he will find cure of all kinds and some discourses and full scale orations

accept modern psychology, the act of telling a dream in the morning (or putting it in writing) is inherently connected to the dream experience. Furthermore, our memory of dreams after awaking is not free from censorship. However, if Aristides in fact put in writing his dreams each morning and kept records of these dreams it would have made it easier for him to hold on to these memories when writing the *Sacred Tales*, both because it is not a memory of the dreams *per se*, but only of their record, and it is more than likely that Aristides came back to these records regularly, even if he lost these records in the late 160s.

The question of the universal validity of modern psychology in general and Freudian-oriented psycho-analysis in particular exceeds the scope of this work and the skills of this author (cf. Fisher and Greenberg (1977) chap. 2). I accept the critical line taken by Stone (1981) 25–26, 40–41; Walde (1999) 121–142; and Price (2004) 228–232 regarding the application of modern theories of psychology in historical research, particularly when it comes to historians' attempts to analyse records of dreams of historical figures (a few examples of such attempts in the field of classical studies are: Dodds (1951) 102–134, and (1965) chap. 2; Michenaud and Dierkens (1976)). However, modern psychology can provide some critical tools for textual analysis in historical research, not the least of which is formulating more accurate questions and setting clearer criteria for prospective answers. It might be of use to quote Peter Gay, who commented in his influential study *Freud for Historians* that, 'Psycho-analysis offers ideas and, in the right setting, with proper self-restraint, even some techniques that may provide un-hoped-for access to popular fantasies, to dreams and slips and other symptomatic acts, and to the defensive tactics that individuals and institutions quite unwittingly employ. It alerts the historians to documents that are useless, silent, and unmeaning without its theories'. (p. 188).

[48] Pearcy (1988) 383.

[49] Pearcy (1988) 384.

[50] Aristid. *Or.* 48.8 K.

> and various visions, and all of the prophecies and oracles about every kind of matter, some in prose, some in verse, and all deserving of a gratitude to the god greater than one might expect.

It is clear, therefore, that the *Sacred Tales* were not written as a medical treatise although they do describe scenes of a medical nature and hold valuable medical information. In sum, an analysis of the narrative form of the *Sacred Tales* leads one to conclude that Aristides' work is *sui generis*,[51] at least from a literary point of view. Whilst it is possible to determine what the *Sacred Tales* are not, it does not seem possible to catalogue them within the familiar taxonomy of Graeco-Roman literature.

Motives for Composition

Whilst the *Sacred Tales* cannot be classified according to any literary genre this does not mean that it is also impossible to determine their *raison d'être*. According to Aristides, the *Sacred Tales* are eulogies to his saviour Asclepius.[52] This is not unprecedented, as we learn from the numerous votive inscriptions in the temples of Asclepius, commemorating the acts of grace the god bestowed upon his sick worshippers.[53] Aristides viewed the very act of recording his dreams as an end in itself: he was following the god's precept. He was not intending to compose a work of history.[54] His self-confessed inability to constrain his dream-record to a chronology proves that at the time of writing Aristides did not conceive of this record as a history of his dreams, his cures or his maladies, but rather as an act of appreciation and gratitude towards the god.[55] The very title of the work, which was inspired by a pronouncement of Asclepius in one of his first revelations, also suggests that the *Sacred Tales* were shaped as a narrative of the miracles performed by Asclepius.[56] One important meaning of a

---

51 At least of the works we now have.

52 Aristid. *Or.* 47.1–4; 48.2–3 K.

53 Quet (1993) 227, argues that the *Sacred Tales* bear a great resemblance to these votive inscriptions. According to Gil Renberg (2003), there are nearly 400 known such votive inscriptions thanking the god for a remedy given via dreams. A general study of these texts is: Veyne (1987) 381–395.

54 Aristid. *Or.* 48.3 K.

55 Aristid. *Or.* 48.3 K. Quoted above, n. 26.

56 In this early predicament Asclepius bestowed his divine approval upon the *Tales* which were already made. When Aristides finally set to compile the *Sacred Tales*, more than two decades later, the memory of this early revelation was still vivid in his mind. It is not unlikely that the memory of this early predicament guided Aristides when entitling his work.

logos in the *Sacred Tales* refers to a single episode (e.g. apparition or god-sent dream), as is evident from *Or.* 48.24; 50.105 K where Aristides refers to previous *logoi*. Weiss argues convincingly that the plural *logoi* in the work's title reflects this notion.[57] On Aristides' first night in the Pergamene Asclepieion the god revealed himself to Zosimus, Aristides' foster-father, in the image of Salvius.[58] Aristides writes:

> ἔφη δ' οὖν ὁ τροφεὺς ὡς ἐν τούτῳ δὴ τῷ σχήματι διαλεχθείη πρὸς αὐτὸν περὶ τῶν λόγων τῶν ἐμῶν ἄλλα τε δή, οἶμαι, καὶ ὅτι ἐπισημήναιτο ὡδὶ λέγων, ἱεροὶ λόγοι.[59]
>
> My foster-father said that in this form he spoke to him, I believe, *concerning my tales* and among other things designated them by name "Sacred Tales".

'Sacred Tales' was a commonly used title in Greek tradition and it usually referred to a sacred legend which called for a rite of special worship, such as a sacred interdiction or a ceremony of initiation. Generally this precept or interdiction was a divine revelation made in the course of an apparition or epiphany.[60] By entitling his work the *Sacred Tales*, Aristides must have had this particular type of work in mind.[61]

The study of the notions of *hieroi logoi* and *hierai bibloi* (ἱεροὶ βίβλοι) was often seen as an aspect of the interrelations between religion and literacy in classical antiquity,[62] and though the use of writing for religious purposes was widespread in Greek and Roman culture there has been a category of writings, generically entitled *Sacred Tales* (*hieroi logoi*) and collected in Sacred Books (*hierai bibloi*), which was 'so marginal that they did not survive, so sublime that they existed only in the religious imagination, or as with some *hierai bibloi*, so secret that they were never committed to writing'.[63] From its first appearance in Herodotus throughout antiquity and the early Christian era, the notion of *hieroi logoi* was accompanied by an aura of mystery.[64] A study of this notion, which existed in the written and unwritten margins of

---

57 Weiss (1998) 16, n. 6.

58 This Salvius was the famous jurist L. Octavius Cornelius Salvius Julianus Aemilianus, *cos. ord.* 148 CE (Behr [1994] 1156). The full name is taken from *ILS* 8973 and A. Merlin, *Inscriptions de la Tunisie* no. 699.

59 Aristid. *Or.* 48.9 K.

60 Cf. Paus. 8.15.2 f.; Festugière (1954) 88.

61 Or, at least, he was conscious that his readership would associate this type of literature with the title of his work.

62 For the widespread use of writings in Greek and Roman culture cf. Harris (1989) 124 f., 170 f.

63 Henrichs (2003) 209. For a typology of *hieroi logoi* see Baumgarten (1998) with the criticism of Henrichs (2003) 209, n. 10.

64 Hdt. 2.81.2; Pl. *Ep.* 7.235 A; Dodds (1965) 40; Festugière (1954) 88, 168; Henrichs (2003) 235.

the sacred, reveals three interconnected couples of notions: the connection between texts and books; the interplay between oral and written traditions; and finally the dynamics between revelation and secrecy.[65] Walter Burkert defines *hieroi logoi* as 'that which is not to be disclosed to the uninitiated, so that a book with such a title is a priori apocryphal'. As Burkert emphasised, *hieroi logoi* are by definition anonymous and whenever we find a *hieros logos* with a name attached to it, it is usually a mythical or quasi legendary figure such as Orpheus and Pythagoras.[66] Martin West defined *hieros logos* as a 'narrative about the gods, or at least a theological exposition of some kind, giving a basis for religious observances'.[67] The implied oral origin of the *hieroi logoi* often served as a reminder of their cultic origin.[68] Recording sacred tales in writing threatened this secrecy and written *hieroi logoi* with an author attached to them were, therefore, often dismissed as frauds.[69] In this respect the *Sacred Tales* of Aristides are a noteworthy exception, but it is an exception which surely intended to bring to mind all that Greek religion associated with this particular genre.

The *Sacred Tales* are not a case of practising *mimesis*.[70] Rather, in composing them Aristides wished to integrate the dreams into his life story, to tell when and under what circumstances each of the dreams was delivered, and to record what were the consequences.[71] More generally Aristides wanted to 'souligner surtout leur caractère divin d'oracles, ou de predictions toujours confirmées par les événements'.[72]

Aristides leads his readership to believe that the chief narrator of the *Sacred Tales* is Asclepius, rather than Aristides himself. Aristides shares with his readers his deliberations about how he should mould the narrative of the *Sacred Tales*, which events should be included, and more generally, his considerations of what was relevant. For example, after describing a pilgrimage he undertook in January, 149 CE to Chios through Clazomenae and Phocaea Aristides' narrative comes to a halt. He then consults Asclepius asking him how the *Tale* should proceed:

---

65 Henrichs (2003) 210, 229.

66 Burkert (1985) 277.

67 West (1983) 13.

68 Henrichs (2003) 239.

69 Burkert (1972) 219 f.

70 Quet (1993) 221. For *mimesis* as a general trend in Greek literature under the Roman Empire see Whitmarsh (2001). If such a work had been Aristides' intention, he would have based it on pre-existing models.

71 Aristid. *Or.* 48.1–4 K.

72 Quet (1993) 221.

ἀλλὰ τὸ ἐντεῦθεν σὸν ἤδη, ὦ δέσποτα, γίγνεται δεῖξαι καὶ παραστῆσαι ὅ τι ἑξῆς λέγοντες καὶ ὅποι τραπόμενοι σοί τ' ἂν κεχαρισμένα ποιοῖμεν καὶ τοῦ λόγου προΐοιμεν ὡς κάλλιστα. πότερα ἐπειδὴ ποταμοῦ καὶ χειμῶνος τοιούτου ὡς κάλλιστα. πότερα ἐπειδὴ ποταμοῦ καὶ χειμῶνος τοιούτου καὶ λουτροῦ μνείαν ἐποιησάμην, ἕτερα ἐφεξῆς τῆς αὐτῆς ἰδέας λέγω καὶ οἷον κατάλογόν τινα λουτρῶν ποιῶμαι χειμερίων τε καὶ θείων καὶ πάντως παραδόξων; ἢ διαλαβὼν τὸν λόγον καί τινα τῶν ἐν μέσῳ διηγήσωμαι; ἢ κράτιστον καὶ τἀν τῷ μέσῳ πάντα ὑπερβάντα ἀποδοῦναι τὸ τέλος τῷ πρώτῳ λόγῳ, πῶς ἔσχε τὰ τῆς χρησμῳδίας τῆς περὶ τῶν ἐτῶν καὶ πῶς ἅπαντα ἀπέβη;[73]

But as to what follows it is your task, O Lord, to make clear and to reveal, by saying what and by turning where, we would do what is gratifying to you and would best continue our tale. Since I have mentioned the river and the terrible winter and the bath, am I next to speak of other things of the same category and am I to compile, as it were, a catalogue of wintry, divine, and very strange baths? Or dividing up my tale, shall I narrate some intermediate events? Or is it best to pass over all the intermediate things and give the conclusion of my first tale,[74] how the oracle about the years held and how everything turned out.

On another occasion, in his encomium to the god, Aristides said that he considered himself to be speaking for Asclepius:

ἐμοὶ γάρ, ὦ δέσποτα Ἀσκληπιέ, πολλὰ καὶ παντοῖα, ὥσπερ ὑπεῖπον, παρὰ σοῦ καὶ τῆς σῆς φιλανθρωπίας γεγένηται, μέγιστον δὲ καὶ πλείστης χάριτος ἄξιον καὶ σχεδὸν ὡς εἰπεῖν οἰκειότατον οἱ λόγοι. τὸ γὰρ τοῦ Πινδάρου μετέβαλες. ἐκείνου μὲν γὰρ ὁ Πὰν τὸν παιᾶνα ὠρχήσατο, ὡς λόγος, ἐγὼ δέ, εἰ θέμις εἰπεῖν, {τῶν σ}ῶν {λόγον} ὑποκριτής εἰμι.[75]

for I have received, O lord Asclepius, as I have said before, many, various gifts from you and your generosity, but the greatest, the one deserving most gratitude, and nearly, one might say, the most becoming is oratory. You have changed what have happened to Pindar. For Pan danced out of his paean, according to the story. I, on the other hand, if it is proper to express it, am an expounder of your words.

Hence, according to Aristides, the very reason for writing the *Sacred Tales* was to pay homage to the god for all the benefactions he granted upon Aristides. Aristides paid this homage by following the god's commands and putting in writing all the things Asclepius had said and done. Aristides, therefore, is merely executing Asclepius' commands.

A second reason, implicit in the text, for writing the *Sacred Tales,* was Aristides' wish to promote himself as an orator. As Downie notes, Aris-

[73] Aristid. *Or.* 48.24 K.
[74] Aristid. *Or.* 48.18 K.
[75] Aristid. *Or.* 42.12 K; with Schwarz' emendation.

tides was very much interested in developing his professional self portrait when writing the *Sacred Tales*.[76] Indeed building upon this idea Holmes has demonstrated that, 'by analyzing how Aristides represents the difficulty of both interpreting and memorializing the body's suffering we can better understand his epic aspirations'.[77] From a different perspective Petsalis-Diomidis has reached similar conclusions, arguing that in the *Sacred Tales* Aristides introduced 'a new social and intellectual elite model and he places religion at its very centre. In the world of the *Hieroi Logoi* the *pepaideumenos* is in close personal touch with the divine'.[78] By ascribing his professional superiority to divine help, which was a common ploy amongst sophists of his day,[79] Aristides argued for a special quality to his work. According to Aristides, in undertaking to practise oratory he was essentially following the medical regimen Asclepius prescribed him.[80] Aristides had already argued that he spoke for the god,[81] and it was therefore Asclepius' will for him to declaim again.[82] Furthermore, during his *cathedra* Asclepius trained Aristides in the art of speaking, mainly through dreams.[83] Hence the quality of his performance was testimony to the god's might. In consequence it would not merely be vanity for another orator to compete with Aristides, it would be absurd.

Indeed in accrediting his professional success to Asclepius, Aristides implicitly suggests that his colleagues lacked this kind of help and therefore could not ascend to his heights. For example, Aristides tells of a visit he made to Smyrna during 167 CE when a rival orator whom he described as a 'certain little Egyptian' (Αἰγυπτίου δέ τινος ἀνθρωπίσκου)[84] was about to declaim. Aristides tells how a god-sent dream instructed him to declaim in the council chamber on the very same day![85] The speech was a great success and the reader is led to believe that Aristides out-performed his rival due to Asclepius' patronage. Another successful oratorical display, which Aristides

---

[76] Downie (2008) 116.
[77] Holmes (2008) 82.
[78] Petsalis-Diomidis (2010) 129.
[79] Aristid. *Or*. 51.3–4 K. Rivalries amongst professional orators were common in the age of the Second Sophistic. Cf. Bowersock (1969) 89–100; Anderson (1986) 43–50, 64–66; Anderson (1993) 35–39; Schmitz (1997) 110–133.
[80] Cf. Aristid. *Or*. 50.14 K.
[81] Aristid. *Or*. 42.13 K.
[82] Aristid. *Or*. 50.14 K.
[83] Aristid. *Or*. 50.25–31 K.
[84] Aristid. *Or*. 51.30 K, surely a derogatory description.
[85] Aristid. *Or*. 51.31 K.

ascribed to the god, took place in Smyrna in January 170 CE.[86] By assigning his success as an orator to Asclepius, Aristides argued that this success was inseparable from the medical care the god bestowed upon him.[87] Asclepius managed his oratorical career just as he saved his body. If one is to believe Aristides, the fact that he was now cured (at the time of writing) must also suggest that his oratory contained something of the divine.

2. The *Sacred Tales* as an Autobiography

Aristides' *Sacred Tales* have also been viewed by modern scholars as an autobiography. Ever since the monumental (and now somewhat dated) work of Misch on the history of autobiography in classical antiquity, who defined the *Sacred Tales* as 'perhaps the strangest autobiographical work of Greek literature',[88] through Boulanger, Dodds and Behr,[89] and up to recent scholars such as Quet, Bompaire, Reardon, Harrison and Petsalis-Diomidis,[90] the *Sacred Tales* have been read as a work with discernable autobiographical characteristics. In a 1993 colloquium on autobiography in classical antiquity, the vast majority of the papers that discussed Greek autobiographies during the high empire considered the *Sacred Tales*.[91] Quet, following Lejeune, accepts the definition of the *Sacred Tales* as a work of autobiography and summarises the chief reasons for doing so: 'Les Discours sacrés correspondent certes à la définition contemporaine la plus générale données par Ph. Lejeune de l'autobiographie, comme "récit rétrospectif en prose qu'une personne réelle fait de sa propre existence, lorsqu'elle met l'accent sur la vie individuelle, en particulier sur l'histoire de sa personnalité"'.[92] Moreover, this inclination to read the *Sacred Tales* as an autobiography may have already found its origin in the works of Aristides' ancient readers. Some very compelling arguments suggest that Libanius shaped his own autobiography on the model of Aristides' *Sacred Tales*.[93]

---

86 Aristid. *Or.* 51.38–41 K.

87 Aristid. *Or.* 51.36 K.

88 Misch (1950) 498.

89 Boulanger (1923) 163; Dodds (1965) 41–45; Behr (1968) 23.

90 Bompaire (1993); Quet (1993); Reardon (1993); Weiss (1998); Harrison (2000); Petsalis-Diomidis (2006a).

91 Bompaire (1993); Quet (1993); Reardon (1993).

92 Quet (1993) p. 215 quoting Lejeune (1975) 14, 44–46. On the general difficulty of classifying the *Sacred Tales* according to a literary genre see Quet, loc. cit., 249–250.

93 Libanius, like many of his contemporary Greek scholars, was a keen admirer of Aristides' work, which led Pack (1947) and Misch (1950) to argue that he shaped his own autobi-

The reading of the *Sacred Tales* as an autobiography often associates them with the votive offerings found in centres of religious healing (particularly in the temples of Asclepius). Such a reading traces in these votive offerings the formative literary mechanism which shaped Aristides' work.[94] More than a century ago, Misch noted that Aristides' inclination to compose the *Sacred Tales* in their particular form must have been encouraged by seeing and reading the numerous votive inscriptions in the temples of Asclepius.[95] Recent scholars tend to agree.[96] Quet argued that Aristides used the same vocabulary to describe his dreams as that which is found in the votive inscriptions from the Asclepieia.[97] The first person voice of the work, alongside a tendency to focus on the experiences of the author and a particular attention to the body, is common amongst votive inscriptions in the various temples of Asclepius.[98] Many of the god's prescriptions found in the *Sacred Tales* also appear in the votive offerings, suggesting that the influence of the votive inscriptions on Aristides' *Sacred Tales* extended to matters of content as well as form.[99] Furthermore, like the votive offerings, the *Sacred Tales* were written with hindsight, after Asclepius' help was secured and a cure was obtained. This hindsight explains the dominant aretalogical narrative of both the *Sacred Tales* and the votive inscriptions. It is a narrative of miracles performed by a god. Bompaire writes:

> Ainsi, l'autobiographie contenue dans les Discours sacrés est une reconstruction a posteriori, où le déroulement des événements est tout à fait secondaire; il est volontiers remplacé par un récit rétrospectif, procédé Romanesque. Quelques thémes sont privilégiés, toujours les mêmes. Ils concernent l'homme des lettres, orateur et poète, ses succès, auprès des grands de ce monde, enfin la vie judiciaire. Et les passages proprement médicaux et

ography on the model of Aristides' *Sacred Tales*. Later scholars continued to look for traces of the *Sacred Tales* in Libanius' autobiography. Norman (1953) and Swain (1996), (2004) disagreed with Pack, but Quet (1993) thinks that there are some discernable traces of the *Sacred Tales* in Libanius' autobiography. Petsalis-Diomidis (2006a) 194, is the latest to adopt this view, following Misch and Pack.

94 Petsalis-Diomidis (2006a) 193–196, with references to most scholars just cited.

95 Misch (1950) 499. Misch's work was originally published in German in 1907.

96 The most comprehensive study of votive inscriptions, which were dedicated after a visual epiphany in either a dream or a daydream is Renberg (2003). In chapter 3, Renberg looks into the evolution of this particular epigraphic pattern.

97 Quet (1993) 240.

98 Cf. LiDonnici (1995), [A4] 92–93; [A8] 96–97; [A15] 104–105; [B5]; Petsalis-Diomidis (2006) 195.

99 Cf. Habicht (1969) n. 139, referring to one Julius Meidias. See also Müller (1987) 194, referring to one Aelius Theon; Petsalis-Diomidis (2006a) 204.

> médico-religieux forment une arétalogie qui souligne certes la puissance d'Asclépios, mais ausi l'éminente qualité de son patient destiné à une apothéose (47.17; 50.50–51 K).[100] Nous sommes appelés à entendre un dialogue intemporal, exemplaire, entre le dieu et le sophiste.[101]

To conclude, the *Sacred Tales* certainly meet the modern definition of an autobiography. They are a work of prose, which focuses on its author's life experiences. Furthermore, the work's form was not an *ex nihilo* creation of Aristides. The imprints of the author's cultural environment are conspicuously present. However, as the work's title suggests, Aristides was not trying in the *Sacred Tales* to compose his autobiography *per se*. The recurrent claims that he composed the *Sacred Tales* as a eulogy, and Aristides' explicit statement that he functioned as a herald of Asclepius,[102] alongside claims that Asclepius was the true author of the *Sacred Tales*,[103] all mark the autobiographical character of the *Sacred Tales* a by-product of aretalogy. One can consider the *Sacred Tales* to be an autobiography because they recorded introspective reflections of an individual upon his own history. However, the autobiographical narrative is just a means to an end. The explicit purpose of the *Tales* is to glorify Asclepius.

3. The Ancient Readers of the *Sacred Tales*

Ancient readers of the *Sacred Tales* did not consider them to be eccentric or unique in either form or content. Philostratus, Sopater, Libanius and Synesius were all familiar with the *Sacred Tales*. Some read the work as a diary and noted that the elaborate record of the dreams in the *Sacred Tales* proved a valuable instrument for an orator. It has also been suggested that Apuleius read the *Sacred Tales*, and 'that Lucius' narrative of religious conversion in Metamorphoses 11 uses and parodies in its detailed comic presentation of a personal religious testament the similar but seriously presented narrative of Aelius Aristides' *Sacred Tales*'.[104] A study of society, medicine and religion in Aristides' *Sacred Tales* will therefore benefit from examining the reactions of ancient readers to the work.

Philostratus, the third-century biographer of the Greek sophists, was familiar with the *Sacred Tales*. He writes that:

---

[100] Cf. Bompaire (1989) 34.
[101] Bompaire (1993) 201–202.
[102] Aristid. *Or*. 42.12 K.
[103] Petsalis-Diomidis (2006) 198–201.
[104] Harrison (2000) 245, and p. 14, n. 16 above.

νοσώδης δὲ ἐκ μειρακίου γενόμενος οὐκ ἠμέλησε τοῦ πονεῖν. τὴν μὲν οὖν ἰδέαν τῆς νόσου καὶ ὅτι τὰ νεῦρα αὐτῷ ἐπεφρίκει, ἐν Ἱεροῖς βιβλίοις αὐτὸς φράζει, τὰ δὲ βιβλία ταῦτα ἐφημερίδων ἐπέχει τινὰ αὐτῷ λόγον, αἱ δὲ ἐφημερίδες ἀγαθαὶ διδάσκαλοι τοῦ περὶ παντὸς εὖ διαλέγεσθαι.[105]

Though sick since childhood he did not refrain from working hard. The nature of his illness and how it made his tendons shiver he himself tells in the Sacred Books. These books provide for him journals of some sort. Journals are excellent teachers for speaking well on any subject.

Philostratus, so it appears, read the *Sacred Tales* essentially as an autobiography and a portrait of an orator. Petsalis-Diomidis noticed that in this passage Philostratus recognised the two central themes of Aristides' *Sacred Tales* to be illness and oratory.[106] He was not critical of their strong religious thread or dubious about their medical content. Likewise, it is implicit in Philostratus' account that Aristides wrote the *Sacred Tales* for publication and that insofar as they are diaries they hold valuable material for those aspiring to an oratorical career. In sum, Philostratus concluded that the *Sacred Tales* were a work worth reading by anyone who wished to become a sophist. Bearing in mind that Philostratus' sophists were also pivotal participants in the Greek civic life during the high empire, Aristides' *Sacred Tales* must have appeared to Philostratus to be an autobiography which would be of interest to anyone wishing to learn about the personal life of a Greek sophist as well as holding a particular attraction for anyone who aspired to join that world.

A different reading of the *Sacred Tales* is that of Sopater, the late fourth century Greek teacher of rhetoric, who mentioned the *Sacred Tales* in his *Prolegomena in Aristidem*. Sopater described the *Sacred Tales* as Aristides' reports of his dreams which brought him miraculous healing.[107] Like many of his contemporary Greek rhetors (cf. Libanius) Sopater was a keen admirer of Aristides' work. His *Prolegomena* was written as 'a zealous advocate of the educational value of Aristides' orations'.[108] It appears from the description of Sopater that he conceived of the *Sacred Tales* as essentially being a work of eulogy. He writes:

οὗτος δὲ ὁ Ἀριστείδης νέος ὢν πικροτάτην λέγεται νενοσηκέναι νόσον· ἐπιληπτικὸν γὰρ αὐτὸν λέγουσι γεγονέναι, καὶ τὸ τῶν λόγων αὐτοῦ διὰ τοῦτο ἠργηκέναι ἐπί τινα χρόνον, εἶτα ἀπελθὼν ἐν Περγάμῳ, ὡς δὴ τοῦ Ἀσκληπιοῦ πολὺ ἐκεῖσε φοιτῶντος,

---

105 Philostr. *VS* 582.
106 Petsalis-Diomidis (2010) 122.
107 Sopater, *Prolegomena* 738D, ed. Lenz (1959) 112.
108 Lenz (1959) 106.

> καὶ παραμείνας χρόνον ἔτυχεν ἰάσεως. ὑπὲρ τούτου ἀμείψασθαι τὴν εὐεργεσίαν βουλόμενος ἔγραψεν ἓξ λόγους τοὺς ἱεροὺς λεγομένους, ἐν οἷς μόνους τοὺς ὀνείρους ἐξηγεῖται, οὓς ἰδὼν ἰάθη.[109]
>
> This Aristides, it is said, became severely ill while still young. They say he became epileptic and, due to that, he stopped working on his speeches for some time. Later he came to Pergamum, on the grounds that Asclepius visited there regularly, and remaining there for a period, he attained cure. In regards to this, wishing to repay the beneficence of the god he composed the six books called 'sacred', in which he expounded only the dreams, the seeing of which cured him.

Another contemporary of Sopater, and admirer of Aristides' work, who was familiar with his *Sacred Tales* was Libanius. As a rhetor Libanius took great interest in Aristides,[110] whom he saw as an exemplary model for Greek Attic speech. Swain, for example, has demonstrated that Libanius' *Or.* 64 (*For the Dancers*) is an *antilogia* of Aristides' speech against the pantomimes.[111] Indeed, Libanius' admiration for Aristides led Boulanger and Pack to argue that the main features of the *Sacred Tales*, namely the long narrative of Aristides' malady, the treatments he underwent and his relationship with Asclepius, were very much present in Libanius' mind when writing his own autobiography (*Or.* 1).[112] Be the level of influence of Aristides' *Sacred Tales* on Libanius' own composition of his autobiography as it may, the late antique rhetor of Antioch was certainly familiar with this work.[113]

In addition to the ancient readers of the *Sacred Tales* who identified autobiographical characteristics in this work, there is at least one ancient reference to the *Sacred Tales* in an oneirocritical context. Synesius, in his treatise *De Insomniis*, used the term 'diary' or 'journal' with direct reference to Philostratus' description of Aristides' *Sacred Tales* in his treatise on dreams. He writes:

> σοφὸν δ' ἂν εἴη καὶ γράφειν τά τε ὕπαρ καὶ ὄναρ ὁράματα καὶ συμπτώματα ... εἰ γὰρ τὰς ἐφημερίδας ὁ Λήμνιος σοφιστὴς ἀγαθὰς εἶναι διδασκάλους φησὶ τοῦ περὶ ἅπαντος εὖ εἰπεῖν.[114]
>
> It would be wise also to write down visions seen and the things that befall us both in dreams and in waking visions ... if indeed the sophist of Lemnos says that journals [of dreams] are good teachers of how to speak well on everything.

---

109 Sopater, *Prolegomena* 738D.
110 Petsalis-Diomidis (2006) 194–196.
111 Swain (2004) 368.
112 Boulanger (1923) 453–454; Pack (1947) 19–20.
113 Cf. Lib. *Ep.* 1534.3.
114 Synesius, *De Insomniis*, 18.2–3.

Synesius also regarded a dream-record such as Aristides' as a valuable aid for rhetoric. Indeed, a later commentator on Synesius' work, Nicephorus Gregoras, said that Synesius kept such a record himself,[115] but produced no evidence for this claim.[116]

It appears that the ancient readers of the *Sacred Tales* all believed they contained credible biographical information regarding Aristides. None of them questioned whether Aristides' malady was genuine. Most read the *Sacred Tales* as a narrative of his illness. Furthermore, there is no indication that any aspect of the work seemed to them as being eccentric or odd. The reports of his medical condition were favourably acknowledged by Philostratus and Sopater. Aristides' devotion to his god was commemorated in Sopater's *Prolegomena* and also by Libanius. Aristides' high regard for his dreams, his understanding of their mechanism and his inclination to interpret them as messages from the gods, were duly noted by Synesius. For these readers, the *Sacred Tales* were not seen as either eccentric or unique, but as a manifestation of contemporary attitudes and experiences.

4. A Narrative of Redemption

Aristides did not commence his writing of the *Sacred Tales* until late in his life because he thought he would not survive his illness.[117] When he did finally start, he chose to describe his illness and the acts of grace Asclepius bestowed upon him in a non-chronological order. This decision means that the narrative of the *Sacred Tales* does not build up tension and avoids the uncertainty of an unknown future. Instead, his readers are aware from the outset that Asclepius saved Aristides and that the *Sacred Tales* tell a story of redemption and salvation by the god.[118] This aretalogical thread is further maintained by Aristides' narrative of his oratorical career. He gave up oratory when he first became ill due to the great physical discomfort he was suffering.[119] Aristides was then summoned by Asclepius to convalesce in his temple in Pergamum. While there the god exhorted him to resume his practice of oratory.[120] This precept was reiterated by his acquaintances. For

115 Synesius, *De Insomniis*, 18.3; Nicephorus Gregoras, *Scholia in Synesii De Insomniis*, p. 632.
116 Behr (1968) 45.
117 Aristid. *Or.* 48.1 K.
118 Aristid. *Or.* 47.1–4 K.
119 Aristid. *Or.* 50.14 K.
120 Aristid. *Or.* 50.14 K.

example the philosopher Euarestus of Crete told Aristides that Asclepius had ordered him to declaim again,[121] and the lyric poet Hermocrates of Rhodes encouraged Aristides to resume declaiming, saying that Asclepius had sent him a dream bearing this message.[122]

Asclepius told Aristides in a dream that, along with Socrates, Demosthenes and Thucydides, *logoi* suited him. Aristides recalled: 'the god commanded me to go to the Temple Stoa, which is at the Theatre, and to offer him [i.e. Asclepius] the very first fruits of these improvised and competitive orations'.[123] Asclepius himself trained Aristides as an orator, mainly through Aristides' dreams.[124] Moreover, Asclepius instructed Aristides to compose hymns not just for him, but for other deities as well.[125] Later Aristides explicitly ascribed his skill and success as an orator to Asclepius:

> ἀλλ' ὅσον μὲν εἰς τὸν θεὸν ἔρχεται τῶν λόγων, ἀνάγκη φράζειν πειρᾶσθαι καὶ μὴ παραλιπεῖν ἐκ τῶν δυνατῶν. ἄτοπον γὰρ εἰ μέν τι τῷ σώματι καὶ κατ' οἶκον ἔδωκεν ἴαμα, διηγεῖσθαι τοῦτ' ἂν καὶ αὐτὸν καὶ ἕτερον, ἐκεῖνα δὲ ἃ ὁμοῦ τὸ σῶμα ἀνίστη, τὴν ψυχὴν ἐπερρώννυ, τοὺς λόγους ηὖξε μετ' εὐδοξίας, ταῦτα δὲ οὑτωσὶ παρελθεῖν σιωπ.[126]
>
> But it is necessary to try to make clear all of my oratorical career that pertains to the god and, as far as I can, to omit nothing of it. For it would be strange if both I and others would recount whatever cure he gave to my body even at home, but would pass by in silence those things which at the same time raised up my body, strengthened my soul and increased the glory of my oratory.

Hence the reader is led to believe that Aristides was saved by Asclepius, but also that his survival itself is an indication of Aristides' professional superiority. By constructing his narrative in this way Aristides achieves two goals: firstly he positions himself as a successor to the great Greek oratorical tradition and as a scholar of distinction, and secondly he defines his practice of oratory as a religious calling.

A narrative of salvation needs to have a starting point of despair. Aristides' report of his long reluctance to write the *Sacred Tales* (because he

---

121 Aristid. *Or.* 50.23 K. The *Sacred Tales* do not tell us how Euarestus learned of Asclepius' command.

122 Εὐάρεστος Κρὴς ... ἔφη προστάξαι τὸν θεὸν αὑτῷ προτρέπειν ἐμὲ πρὸς τοὺς λόγους ... 'Euarestus of Crete ... and he said that the god commanded him to exhort me to take up rhetoric ...'. Ibid.

123 καὶ τό γε σφόδρα πρῶτον ἀπάρξασθαί με ἐκέλευεν ἑαυτῷ προσελθόντα εἰς τὴν στοὰν τοῦ ἱεροῦ τὴν πρὸς τῷ θεάτρῳ τῶν αὐτοσχεδίων δὴ τούτων λόγων καὶ ἀγωνιστικῶν. Aristid. *Or.* 50.15 K.

124 Aristid. *Or.* 50.25–31 K.

125 Aristid. *Or.* 50.39 K.

126 Aristid. *Or.* 51.36 K.

expected death) fulfils this need.[127] Whilst Aristides was in the pit of despair, after returning sick from Rome in the winter of 144 CE, Asclepius made his first revelation to him in the warm springs near Pergamum.[128] Asclepius addressed Aristides in his dream, ordering him to go unshod, 'and I cried out in my dream, as if in a waking state and after I had accomplished the orders of the dream: "great is Asclepius! The order is accomplished"' (ἀνυπόδητόν τε γὰρ προελθεῖν ἐπέταξε καὶ ἐβόων δὴ ἐν τῷ ὀνείρατι ὡς ἂν ὕπαρ τε καὶ ἐπ' ὀνείρατι τετελεσμένῳ, μέγας ὁ 'Ασκληπιὸς, τετέλεσται τὸ πρόσταγμα).[129] This is the moment of recognition of the power of the god.[130] It is also a transition phase in the narrative where hope replaces despair. Having woken up, and understanding the dream as an invitation to travel from Smyrna to the Pergamene Asclepieion, Aristides goes without delay 'with good fortune' (μετὰ τῆς ἀγαθῆς τύχης).[131]

It is typical in salvation narratives for there to be a clear moment when the protagonist makes a conscious submission to the god.[132] Aristides opens the first *Sacred Tale* by declaring his decision 'to submit to the god, truly as to a doctor, and to do in silence whatever he wishes' (ταῦτ' οὖν ἐνθυμούμενος ἐγνώκειν παρέχειν ὡς ἀληθῶς ὥσπερ ἰατρῷ τῷ θεῷ σιγῇ ποιεῖν ὅ τι βούλεται).[133] Furthermore, the fact that Aristides was alive and in good health more than two decades after initially falling ill, and that he then followed Ascelpius' precept to compose the *Sacred Tales*, demonstrates that he was still a devout worshipper. It also demonstrates that he was saved by the god.

Aristides' sense of security and faith in the god had been established during his first night at the temple when the god appeared to Zosimus, Aristides' foster-father, discussing Aristides' *Tales* 'and among other things designated them by name "The Sacred Tales"'.[134] In this way Aristides' narrative of salvation becomes interwoven with his career as an orator and an author. From this point onwards Aristides' rhetoric will have a special meaning in the *Sacred Tales* as an inherent component of Asclepius' prescription and is designated as having a medical role.

---

127 Aristid. *Or.* 48.1 K.

128 Aristid. *Or.* 48.7 K.

129 Aristid. *Or.* 48.7 K.

130 Weiss (1998) and Harrison (2000) read the *Sacred Tales* as a narrative of conversion. If one is to accept their interpretation, this is the turning point in which Aristides converted to the cult of Asclepius.

131 Ibid.

132 Cf. James (1982) 4.

133 Aristid. *Or.* 47.4 K.

134 ἔφη δ' οὖν ὁ τροφεὺς ὡς ἐν τούτῳ δὴ τῷ σχήματι διαλεχθείη πρὸς αὐτὸν περὶ τῶν λόγων τῶν ἐμῶν ἄλλα τε δὴ, οἶμαι, καὶ ὅτι ἐπισημήναιτο ὡδὶ λέγων, ἱεροὶ λόγοι. Aristid. *Or.* 48.9 K.

Once having gained the assurance that Asclepius was his protector, Aristides lost all fear. He embarked on a sea journey from Clazomenae to Phocaea, under Asclepius' command, and was nearly shipwrecked. However, unlike the rest of the passengers and seamen, Aristides was confident, saying only 'O Asclepius!' (ὦ Ἀσκληπιέ).[135] His faith allowed Aristides to comprehend such adversity as being part of the god's plan and therefore inevitable: it had been his fate for this misfortune to occur. He would therefore have to undergo such tribulations in order that 'my fate would be fulfilled' (ἐν γὰρ τούτῳ τελεῖσθαι τὰ ἀναγκαῖα).[136] Hence the shipwreck, which involved real danger, seemed wonderful to Aristides because 'we also knew it was indeed he who saved us from the sea too'.[137] On another occasion, when Asclepius commanded Aristides to bathe in an icy river, Aristides complied wholeheartedly, crying 'great is Asclepius'.[138] A sense of redemption stayed with Aristides for the rest of the day and he reported that he felt warm and healthy.[139]

The impression that the *Sacred Tales* form a narrative of salvation is augmented by the rhetoric Aristides employed. By having Asclepius tell his story, as if the *Sacred Tales* are Asclepius' and not his own, Aristides persuades the reader that his story is part of a greater divine plan. It is the task of Asclepius, for example, to show how the prophecy about Aristides' time of death turned out to be true.[140]

Perhaps one of the most interesting and detailed expositions of Aristides' faithfulness and dependence upon Asclepius can be seen in his dream from the end of March, 146 CE. In the course of the dream the god predicts that Aristides will die in two days 'and this was inevitable' (ἔφη χρῆναι τελευτᾶν εἰς τρίτην ἡμέραν, καὶ ταῦτα ἀναγκαίως ἔχειν).[141] It was possible for this prediction to be overturned, however, because Aristides followed to the letter the commands of Asclepius, which included a pilgrimage, a sacrifice and the requirement that he cut off a part of his body (although this was later lessened to the offering of a ring).[142] The scene ends with a sense of total submission of Aristides to Asclepius: 'after this it is possible to imagine how

---

135 Aristid. *Or.* 48.12 K.

136 Aristid. *Or.* 48.13 K.

137 οὖ δὴ καὶ ἔγνωμεν ὅτι κἀκ τοῦ πελάγους ἄρα αὐτὸς ὁ σεσωκὼς ἦν. Aristid. *Or.* 48.14 K.

138 μέγας ὁ Ἀσκληπιός. Aristid. *Or.* 48.21 K.

139 Aristid. *Or.* 48.21–22 K.

140 Aristid. *Or.* 48.24 K.

141 Aristid. *Or.* 48.26 K.

142 Aristid. *Or.* 48.26–28 K.

we were disposed, and into what kind of harmony the god again brought us. We fared in regards to all this as if in an initiation ritual, with good hope attending us along with fear'.[143] This description is typical of accounts of religious encounters. In his seminal study of the *Varieties of Religious Experience*, William James commented that in the religious life acts of surrender and sacrifice are promoted. Religion is viewed as giving meaning to difficult or troubling events or circumstances.[144] It is common in the pages of religious biography to find that episodes of hardship or challenges to faith are described as life-altering. James notes that many a religious person has the recollection of a particular crisis in which a direct vision or perception of the god swept in and overwhelmed the languor of a more orderly belief.[145] Seen in this light, the medical theme in the *Sacred Tales* is subject to an overall religious meta-narrative.[146]

The narrative-thread running throughout the *Sacred Tales* is Aristides' salvation by the god.[147] It acts as a unifying element, bringing together the multitude of subjects and periods of time collected in this work. This general theme of salvation by Asclepius is then augmented by explicit prophecies, such as the prediction of the oracle in Colophon that 'Asclepius will cure and heal your disease in honour of the famous city of Telephus';[148] or a dream in which the god told Aristides he has been cured.[149] At one point when concluding a story about a dream that took place in the Pergamene Asclepieion during 146 CE, Aristides decided to 'finish the story, and add how the oracle concerning the years [i.e. the prophecy that he had seventeen years left to live] turned out'.[150] Aristides explains that throughout this time

---

143 τὸ δὴ μετὰ τοῦτο ἔξεστιν εἰκάζειν ὅπως διεκείμεθα, καὶ ὁποίαν τινὰ ἁρμονίαν πάλιν ἡμᾶς ἡρμόσατο ὁ θεός. σχεδὸν γὰρ ὥσπερ ἐν τελετῇ περὶ πάντα ταῦτα διήγομεν, παρεστώσης ἅμα τῷ φόβῳ τῆς ἀγαθῆς ἐλπίδος. Aristid. *Or*. 48.28 K.

144 James (1982) 51–52.

145 James (1982) 65.

146 A meta-narrative is a global narrative which orders and explains knowledge and experience.

147 Salvation in a sense that due to Asclepius' acts of grace Aristides is still alive. Aristides explicitly made this claim in a speech he delivered during his stay in the Asclepieion. He argued that contrary to the likelihood of the circumstances, he was alive, having escaped at different times through various kinds of consolation and advice on the part of the god, from things no doctor knew what to call, to say nothing of cure, nor had seen befall the nature of man. Aristid. *Or*. 2.67–68 L-B.

148 Ἰήσεταί σε νοῦσον ἠδ' ἀκέσσεται Ἀσκληπιὸς, πόλισμα Τηλέφου κλυτὸν τιμῶν. Aristid. *Or*. 49.12 K.

149 Aristid. *Or*. 49.5 K.

150 Φέρε δὴ τὸν ἐξ ἀρχῆς ἀποδῶμεν λόγον, καὶ συνάψωμεν ὡς ἔσχε τὰ τῆς χρησμῳδίας τῆς περὶ τῶν ἐτῶν. Aristid. *Or*. 48.37 K.

Asclepius was his saviour, granting him his continued existence.[151] When his appointed time to die came the plague was raging in the province of Asia. Aristides and many of his household were infected. However, Aristides was saved after Athena instructed him in a vision to persevere.[152] On the day Aristides recovered his favourite foster-child died. An oracle later confirmed Aristides' feelings that the girl's death was not without divine intervention.[153] Aristides saw an inherent connection between the two events, and he formed them in his account into one coherent narrative of salvation. Aristides explains: 'thus I had my life up to this time as a bounty from the gods, and after this, I was given a new life through the gods, and this, as it were, kind of exchange occurred [i.e. his life for the life of the girl]'.[154] Aristides concluded: 'and thus took place the prediction concerning my years, and my later sickness, which agreed with this, and the divine manifestations pertaining to these things'.[155] This episode is therefore indicative of Aristides' conviction in the redemptive power of the god and that the *Sacred Tales* are an account of faith.

Conclusion

This first chapter has clarified a number of issues concerning the composition of the *Sacred Tales*, notably their time of writing, the nature of the source-material used and, perhaps most importantly, Aristides' motives for their composition and publication. The chapter has also analysed the *Sacred Tales* by reviewing their impact on their ancient readership. The study has concurred with scholars such as Petsalis-Diomidis by pointing out that the text was an act of self-presentation and cannot be read literally. It has been demonstrated, too, that the *Sacred Tales* have many traits of autobiography

151 Ibid.

152 Aristid. *Or.* 48.42 K. An apparition of Athena, of all deities, must have acted as a clear reference to the well-known apparition of Athena to Achilles in the first book of the *Iliad.* As in the Homeric epos the appearance and actions of the goddess of wisdom led the heroes to make the right decision. Achiles refrained from killing Agammenon and Aristides wisely followed the prescribed regimen of the goddess. Furthermore, like in the Homeric epos, Athena appears to Aristides alone. (Aristid. *Or.* 48.41 K.)

153 Aristid. *Or.* 51.21 K.

154 οὕτω τόν τε ἄχρι τούτου χρόνον δωρεὰν ἔσχον παρὰ τῶν θεῶν καὶ μετὰ τοῦτο ἀνεβίων ὑπὸ τοῖς θεοῖς καί τις οἷον ἀντίδοσις αὕτη συνέβη. Aristid. *Or.* 48.44 K.

155 Καὶ τὰ μὲν τῆς προρρήσεως τῆς περὶ τῶν ἐτῶν καὶ τῆς ὕστερον ἀσθενείας εἰς τοῦτο συμβάσης καὶ τῶν περὶ ταῦτα ἐπιφανειῶν οὕτως ἔσχεν. Aristid. *Or.* 48.45 K.

and Aristides' own experiences are their sole concern. The method he chose to describe his story, namely the use of the first person narrative, is further evidence of the autobiographical nature of the work. In addition it has been shown how the *Tales* are an account of faith and the theme of salvation runs throughout them. However, the *Sacred Tales* can also be viewed as part of the corpus of work of the writers of so-called Second Sophistic, sharing their use of pure Attic Greek and, more generally, the cultural domain in which they operated. While acknowledging both the subjectivity of the *Sacred Tales* and the rhetorical devices Aristides employed, the following chapters will further contextualize the text by examining how far it is possible to accept the testimony of the *Sacred Tales* as authoritative and representative of their social context, particularly in the fields of medicine and religion.

CHAPTER TWO

SOCIETY, DISEASE AND MEDICINE IN THE *SACRED TALES* OF ARISTIDES

Introduction

The *Sacred Tales* of Aelius Aristides often discuss medical issues. These include Aristides' own descriptions of his malady and the appeals for health-care he made to physicians and gods; the medical treatments he underwent and the institutions which provided it; more general descriptions of the medical care which was offered in the Pergamene Asclepieion; and valuable contributions to a prosopography of contemporary physicians. The *Sacred Tales* can therefore provide a historian of ancient medicine with a valuable opportunity to examine the subject, particularly from the patient's point of view. The history of medicine, both as a history of ideas as well as a social history of medicine,[1] has only limited first hand evidence about medicine during the high empire. Detailed accounts of the experiences of the sick themselves are exceptionally rare.[2] Information about the place of medicine in society and about the comprehension of medicine by laymen, rather than professional practitioners of medical care, is also scarce. Basic questions concerning the attitude of society to its sick and their place in society are still inadequately studied. Furthermore, a history of the sick themselves, which asks how they conceived of their illness; what they perceived as a medical procedure; and whom they deemed as authoritative in providing health-care, has not yet been written. More generally, the questions of whether a medical discourse existed at all, and if so, how this discourse was anchored in social institutions can benefit greatly from an

[1] The social history of medicine looks into the development of social trends in relation to medicine; Jordanova (1995); D. Porter (1995).

[2] See here the provocative study by Perkins of pain and narrative representation in the early Christian era. Perkins demonstrated how during this time pre-existing models of bodily representation have changed. Perkins found in the *Sacred Tales* evidence for embracing bodily suffering and transforming it into power of transcendence. Perkins also found parallels to this tendency in Gal. *Prog.*, and in M.Ant. *Med.*, as well in the work of Epictetus and Seneca [Perkins (1995) chaps. 3, and 7].

exploration of the *Sacred Tales*. This chapter will therefore look into disease and medicine in the *Sacred Tales* of Aelius Aristides.

After initially falling ill in the early 140s, Aristides made considerable efforts to comprehend his medical condition and to secure treatment. He consulted various health-care providers, and also sought divine help. He followed the regimens of physicians and gods, which included medicinal dietary habits, the use of drugs and some elaborate procedures of cleansing. In addition, Aristides undertook sacred pilgrimages and even surgical measures. In this chapter I will ask what Aristides' concepts of medicine and disease were, what they meant to him, and how the society in which he lived influenced his understanding of these notions. Next I will examine the attitude of society towards disease, as an abstract notion and in relation to the sick themselves, that is depicted in the *Sacred Tales*. I will then proceed to consider the nature of medicine in the world of the *Sacred Tales*, both as an explanatory model and as a social institution.

The autobiographical description of being sick and seeking medical help which Aristides left in his *Sacred Tales* is unique both in its form and content. In this work Aristides described his intimate relationship with Asclepius over the course of almost thirty years. He gives a record of more than 130 dreams that the god sent him and which mostly offered advice in respect of his poor health. Aristides also included in the *Sacred Tales* many of his consultations with a range of other health-care providers (including physicians and priests) and the various treatments he underwent. It is therefore necessary to address the question of whether Aristides' description can be seen as representative of the experience of being ill in Graeco-Roman times. Moreover, because the meaning of medicine changes throughout time and across cultures, and because what falls under the remit of medicine in certain circumstances lies elsewhere in others, a corroborative study of ancient medicine, classical approaches to the interpretation of dreams and the relevant aspects of the cult of Asclepius are all necessary in order to contextualise the *Sacred Tales*.

Such a comparative study of disease and medicine in the world of the *Sacred Tales* benefits from a wide range of relevant evidence. In addition to the *Sacred Tales* themselves, I will draw on medical works, from the Hippocratic corpus to the work of Galen; ancient treatises on dreams; and archaeological evidence, such as the votive inscriptions from centres of religious healing and the temples of Asclepius themselves. All these sources are likely to make a significant contribution to establishing the framework in which the *Sacred Tales* belong. The wide spectrum of corroborating evidence will be used to examine different aspects of Aristides' experiences of falling ill and seeking medical help. The medical works will be used to examine whether Aristides' choices of treatment-options were representative of his age and whether his manner of conceptualizing his medical condition embodied common modes of thinking in Graeco-Roman medicine. In addition, similar questions will be asked regarding Aristides' approach to dreams. Votive inscriptions and other archaeological evidence from the temples of Asclepius will constitute a background for looking into the religious aspects of Aristides' understanding of his illness and pursuit of therapy.

From a methodological point of view, the most challenging aspect of this study of medicine and disease in Aristides' *Sacred Tales* will be to locate Aristides' thoughts and deeds within the more general belief system that prevailed in his world.[3] Realizing the inappropriateness of subjecting Aristides' habits to modern understandings of human physiology and medicine and the distinction between science and religion,[4] while avoiding the trap of absolute relativism, calls for particular attention to the use of these notions in Aristides' world and to the difficulties of translating one conceptual scheme into another. In the first section of the chapter I therefore address these issues of methodology by discussing in more general terms the notion of a 'health-care system' as a conceptual scheme, using anthropological and sociological tools. I then specifically focus upon the notions of medicine and the dream-mechanism in Graeco-Roman world. The second section of the chapter looks into the sick, medicine and physicians in the world of the *Sacred Tales*. Finally, in the last section, I endeavour to unite these different investigative strands within a history of Aelius Aristides' medical condition.

---

[3] On the notion of 'belief' in Greek religion see Harrison (2007).

[4] For an analysis of the modern view of the body in general, and of the mechanistic nature of medicine in particular see the stimulating work of Helman (1984) who explores the meanings of health and disease, and the symbolic significance of therapies, from the viewpoint of the sick person and the community.

1. The Graeco-Roman Health-Care System[5]

Towards a Definition of a Medical Discourse[6]

The measures Aristides took to fight his illness might seem extreme to a modern reader. However, extremity is both contextually and culturally determined. The work of Arthur Kleinman, an American physician, psychiatrist, and anthropologist emphasised the 'inner structure' of health-care systems.[7] In his work Kleinman defined the health-care system as a concept, not as an entity; he saw the health-care system as a conceptual model held by the researcher. Scholars, he noted, derive their understanding of this model by learning how the actors in a particular social setting think about health-care. Their beliefs about sickness, the measures they take to tackle it and their expectations and evaluations of the various types of treatment available to them help scholars form a model of the health-care system. Such a model is also determined by examining the way people act towards and make use of the components in this system. The health-care system includes people's beliefs and patterns of behaviour, although they are not necessarily fully aware of all of them when operating within such a system.[8] Those beliefs and practices are regulated by social rules. Hence health-care systems comply with Clifford Geertz's definition of a cultural system: they are both maps 'for' and 'of' a special area of human behaviour.[9] As Kleinman has noted: 'In the same sense in which we speak of religion or language or kinship as cultural systems, we can view medicine as a cultural system, a system of symbolic meanings anchored in particular arrangements of social institutions and patterns of interpersonal interactions'.[10]

---

[5] It is justifiable and heuristic to describe the entire range of health-related activities in the Graeco-Roman world (or any other society) as a *system* of health-care because it is equivalent to a cultural system. This means that the Graeco-Roman health-care system was guided by a set of rules (social, scientific, religious metaphysical etc.) which directed members of society how to use this system (e.g. they guided Aristides how to conceive of his pathologies; offered him a range of health-care providers and a spectrum of medical solutions). These rules can also be inferred by an observer (either internal or external) who, in turn, can understand from watching the particular actors within the health-care system, what are the rules that guide it.

[6] My whole approach to this subject owes much to the stimulating work of Kleinman (1980).

[7] Kleinman (1980).

[8] Kleinman (1980) 25–26.

[9] Geertz (1973) 3–30.

[10] Kleinman (1980) 24.

The health-care system integrates the health-related components of a society. In the words of Kleinman, these include 'patterns of beliefs about the causes of illness; norms of governing choice and evaluation of treatment; socially legitimate statuses, roles, power relationships, interaction settings, and institutions'.[11] Because both patients and healers are parts of this system they cannot be understood outside of this contextual framework. A survey of the Graeco-Roman health-care system is therefore pertinent to a history of Aristides' disease because the health-care system encompasses all knowledge, practices, and authorities which a given society associates with medicine.

According to Kleinman there are four key issues that need to be considered here: the health-care system itself, the dichotomy between two aspects of sickness (illness and disease),[12] the explanatory model, and the semantic network. The clinical phenomena are to be seen as an integral part of the health-care system. He states: 'In every culture, illness, the response to it, individuals experiencing and treating it, and the social institutions relating to it are all systematically interconnected'.[13] In other words, both patients and healers should be seen in one holistic manner in the health-care system, with its symbolic meaning and particular ways of allocating and arranging of power.[14] This system is anchored in institutions and patterns of interpersonal interaction. A health-care system 'is both the result of and the condition for the way people react to sickness in local, social, and cultural settings, for how they perceive, label and explain, and treat sickness'.[15]

Anthropologists have suggested that despite the many variances between health-care systems they nonetheless share one set of 'core clinical functions'. These encompass:

1. The cultural construction of illness as a psychological experience.
2. The establishment of general criteria to guide the health-care seeking process and to evaluate treatment-approaches that exist prior to and independently from individual episodes of sickness.
3. The management of particular illness episodes through communicative operations, such as labelling and explaining.

---

[11] Kleinman (1980) 24.

[12] 'Illness' is a response to a certain physical or psychological symptoms. 'Disease' is the reformulation of illness by the healer.

[13] Kleinman (1980) 24.

[14] Nijhuis (1995) 52.

[15] Kleinman (1980) 26.

4. Healing activities *per se*, which include all types of therapeutic intervention, from drugs and surgery to psychotherapy, supportive care, and healing rituals.
5. The management of therapeutic outcomes, including cure, treatment failure, recurrence, chronic illness, impairment, and death.[16]

Medical anthropologists rely on the concept of the 'explanatory model' and the 'semantic network'. Illness and disease themselves are explanatory models of sickness.[17] The work of Thomas Kuhn, an American philosopher and sociologist of science, stressed the inherent role played by metaphysics in any kind of scientific research.[18] Kuhn argued that no phenomenon is explicable without the existence of theory and methodology.[19] He uses the notion of 'paradigms' to describe conceptual schemes in which any scientific pursuit such as medicine takes place. By shifting his centre of interest from the individual scientist to the community in which a scientist operates Kuhn was also able to demonstrate just how effectively these paradigms manage scientific enterprises. A paradigm provides the practitioner of any particular branch of science a model from which practice can emerge. In the case of ancient medicine such practices and the traces of a particular metaphysics can be detected, for example, in the use medicine made of dreams. Gaining knowledge of these models and becoming familiar with the paradigm as a whole is a preliminary stage for any prospective practitioner wishing to establish himself as a member of a scientific community, such as physicians and dreams-interpreters.

In the field of classics, Tamsyn Barton has demonstrated that by the process of learning a paradigm (Barton focused on three case-studies: ancient astrology, physiognomics and medicine) and by moulding this process of learning into a master-pupil relationship, it became meaningful to talk about 'knowledge' in these disciplines.[20] Those sharing a paradigm also share methods and practices of scientific work and enable the continuation of a given scientific tradition.[21] This social mechanism of regulating scientific activity means that science is interwoven within a discourse of

---

16 Quoted from Kleinman (1980) 71–72.
17 Nijhuis (1995) 54.
18 Kuhn (1962) 7.
19 Kuhn (1962) 25.
20 Barton (1994). For a study of physiognomic as a science, which is both useful for medicine and for predicting the future in the second century CE see Swain (2007).
21 Kuhn (1962) 21.

power. Barton argues that what becomes defined as 'knowledge' is a result of 'power', and in turn those who are seen as possessors of 'knowledge' may participate in power. By focusing our attention on the way society regulates every scientific activity by assigning each of these activities to its appropriate paradigm (e.g. medicine, interpretation of dreams etc.) we can learn how each society develops agreed criteria to distinguish proper praxis in each of these fields from heresies. In the case of ancient medicine, the explanatory model which paradigms provide can help to explain aetiology, time and mode of symptoms, pathophysiology, course and cause of sickness, as well as treatment. Hence in the context of medicine one can speak of a semantic network of illness, which means that illness is, in the words of Nijhuis, 'a configuration of concepts, symbols and experiences, firmly embedded in culture, the meaning of which becomes clear in interaction'.[22]

A history of Aristides' sickness, his response to it, and the measures he took to combat it, contains a dialectical tension between his private and very personal experience of sickness and the socially-organised responses to disease available to him in the Graeco-Roman health-care system. In other words, though the experiences Aristides recorded in the *Sacred Tales* are private and very much his own, they do reflect general patterns of power-structures both by depicting figures of authority in the field of health-care and by marking these figures as carriers of 'knowledge'. As we shall see, the health-care system Aristides turned to had three chief characteristics: the first of these is that second century CE medical thought and institutions had yet to divorce themselves from religion; a second characteristic is that a considerable proportion of medicine's 'set texts' were also an indispensable part of the more general Greek *paideia* and therefore inseparable from the particular shape of Greek identity in the age of Aristides; the third distinctive characteristic of Graeco-Roman medicine is that as a result of a pre-scientific (in its modern sense) frame of thought and before the introduction of experiment-based science and the principle of trial and error, Graeco-Roman medicine lacked a notion of scientific linear progress. New knowledge was not superior to old knowledge and recent medical ideas and thoughts did not render older ones obsolete. Moreover, because the Graeco-Roman health-care system is a cultural system, chronology has a different function here. We are not in search of a genealogy of ideas but the way in which a web of ideas, already established, operated on the actors within

[22] Nijhuis (1995) 54.

it. The fact that the Hippocratic Corpus, for example, was completed five centuries before Aristides' day did not diminish its force in this medical discourse. Likewise, the particular role of *paideia* in the world of Aristides placed classical authors in a privileged position within this system. The Graeco-Roman health-care system did not arrange ideas by their date of arrival but by their medical authority. In this world new was not necessarily better than old.

In this chapter I will use these critical notions in order to learn what can be said about medicine, religion and the interconnections between them in the world of Aelius Aristides as depicted in his *Sacred Tales*. I will also try to learn how the *Sacred Tales* and the person who composed them were seen in this world and whether they can be viewed as being representative of their age.

Medicine in the Graeco-Roman World

As both social anthropology and the history of medicine have convincingly shown in recent years, ideas about disease and what it affects are anything but simple cross-cultural universals.[23] In the Graeco-Roman world those who were seen as competent to help the sick varied from charismatic healers, who cured by a word, a prayer or a healing touch of a hand, through to those with experience in setting fractures or dislocations, to those who could call on the authority of a scholarly tradition.[24] The spectrum between learned and popular tradition—in many cases a difference of degree rather than kind—also exists in the field of medicine, where literacy was easily translated into power and authority.[25] Trying to comprehend disease leads to ideas of the self, of the human body and the way it operates. As Ruth Padel has demonstrated, in ancient Greece the connection between body and mind was highly relevant when it came to apprehending disease.[26]

It is also necessary to consider the role played by ideas of causation and responsibility in ancient medicine, including theodicy.[27] Such an under-

---

[23] Lloyd (2003) 1. A more general approach to the history of medicine, mainly from a social point of view is Amundsen (1996); the articles collected by Bates (1995) look into knowledge and the medical tradition from the point of view of intellectual history. Good (2000) is a stimulating discussion of medicine, rationality and experience from the point of view of the anthropologist.

[24] Lloyd (2003) 2.

[25] Seminal here is Goody (1977).

[26] Padel (1992).

[27] Already in the *Iliad* one finds Apollo causing and curing the plague sent on the Achaean

standing is paramount for deciphering the inner structure of the Graeco-Roman health care system. The relevance of the gods raises the issue of pollution and purity. It was widely held in antiquity that pollution could cause disease. Purification was therefore expected to deal with both disease and pollution.[28] Purification may be a matter of ritual cleansing, prayer and sacrifice, and a means of atoning for offences of a religious nature.[29] The Hippocratic treatise *On the Sacred Disease* demonstrates how common it was to address epilepsy by means of purification, and this was also true of madness.[30] However, the attack made by the Hippocratic author of the *Sacred Disease* was not directed against temples and shrines *per se*, but against those who claimed ability to drive out demons and compel the gods to help by means of charms and chants.[31] It is a criticism of Theophrastus' superstitious man rather than an attempt to exclude the gods from the field of medicine.[32] Five centuries later Plutarch, another fierce opponent of superstitions and their damaging effect, reiterated Theophrastus' accusations against the superstitious men who ignored the advice of their physicians,[33] much like the author of *On the Sacred Disease*. Plutarch, however, was himself a religious person and a Delphic priest who often spoke favourably about purgation.[34] It appears that neither Plutarch nor his readership saw any fault or sign of eccentricity in his doing so. Purification as a

army. Artemis is also said to have punished a city unjust to its citizens and foreigners with a plague on its herds and blight on its corps, early death of young men and stillborn babies, or cripples (Call. *Hec.* 3.122 ff.). Hera is reported to have driven Proitos' daughters mad. Demeter caused a global famine when her beloved daughter was abducted. For further examples see Mattes (1970) 36–49. Furthermore, consultation of the Delphic oracles in regards to cures for plagues habitually took the form 'to which of the gods should we sacrifice to obtain relief?' [Furley and Bremer vol. i (2001) 207–208].

28 Hippoc. *Flat.* 14.48 = Loeb 2: 250; *Morb. Sacr.* 4.53= Loeb 4:148; Padel (1992); Parker (1983) 220.

29 Moulinier (1952); Douglas (1966); Parker (1983).

30 Cf. Ar. *V.* 118.

31 For an authoritative discussion of the Hippocratic treatise *On the Sacred Disease* see the annotated edition of Jouanna (2003). See also Temkin (1971) 2–27; Grmek (1983) 69–71; Wöhlers (1999); Laskaris (2002). Also relevant are the comments in Hippoc. *Vict.* 87, where the author accepts the validity of prayers alongside medical counselling. Furthermore, he claims to have gained all his knowledge about healthy diet from the god (Hippoc. *Vict.* 93). The two treatises are commonly held to have been written by the same author, cf. Jouanna (1999) 374–375.

32 Theophr. *Char.* 16.

33 Plut. *Mor.* 168b–c.

34 Cf. Plut. *Rom.* 21.4; 21.9, 10; *Num.* 19.5; *Cam.* 20.5; *Quomodo adolescens poetas audire debeat*, 19 f.; 51a; *De tuenda sanitate praecepta*, 134a.

means of tackling illness was also common in Rome.[35] Therefore pollution and purification were inherent features of the Graeco-Roman health-care system. The categories of religion and ritual on the one hand and medicine and science on the other were far from distinct.

Even the Hippocratic corpus,[36] in many respects the rationalistic alternative to temple medicine, to a large extent followed existing traditions rather than establishing new ones *ex nihilo*.[37] At most stages in the history of the Western medical tradition inherited images from earlier times integrated with contemporary views, local religions, and existing social structures in order to create and control an image of disease. Post-Hippocratic Greek medical thought was not free from earlier traditions such as those of Homer and Empedocles.[38] Moreover, as the speech of Eryximachus in Plato's *Symposium* exemplified, even after Hippocratic notions entered Greek intellectual discourse pre-Hippocratic notions did not disappear.[39] However, sixth and early fifth century healers could act, like Empedocles, as roving shamans, rendering all clear distinction between medicine and religion irrelevant. Later developments brought significant changes and from 350 BCE onwards it is possible to speak of 'orthodoxy within medicine'.[40] This did not mean, however, that doctors rejected all explanations and therapies that fell into the category of religion. According to Plato, the healing activities prescribed by the physician and by the sacred healer were very similar. Purification, as a case in point, was prescribed by physicians and religious healers alike. It was up to the patient to determine the act's true meaning.[41] As noted in more general terms by Kleinman, the cultural construction of illness is a key factor in shaping the health care system. Thus, the room left in the Greek world for the sick to perceive their condition in both physical and metaphysical terms discloses a particular type of understanding of the nature of illness. In turn, such an understanding marked particular types of health care providers as likely to be able to assist the sick. In this respect

35 Tib. 1.5.11–12; Ov. *Ars*. 2.329 f.

36 The fact that the Hippocratic corpus reached its canonical form almost five centuries before Aristides composed his *Sacred Tales* does not diminish its relevance to a contextual study of Aristides. The Hippocratic corpus was still pertinent in the second century CE, as we learn, amongst other sources, from the work of Galen.

37 Parker (1983) 213.

38 Padel (1992) 50.

39 Pl. *Sym*.185e6–188e5; Cf. Craik (2010).

40 Nutton (2004) 113.

41 Pl. *Cra*. 405a–b.

the pivotal place of *katharsis* (κάθαρσις) in the Hippocratic corpus is revealing.[42] The body according to the Hippocratic view is a carrier whose purity is naturally maintained by a natural cycle of purification.[43] When the body is healthy this process proceeds without any need for help from the outside, but when for some reason or other the bodily balance is interrupted outside help is needed.[44] This is effected by the Hippocratic physician through a purgative drug (φάρμακον).[45] The relation between a purification which is medical and one which is religious is hard to define. The two methods shared a common ideal of purity, which was both physical and metaphysical.[46]

Greek literature, inscriptions, and archaeological remains present many accounts of illness and recuperation, usually written or engraved after the healing was accomplished (e.g. the *Sacred Tales* of Aristides or the votive inscriptions from the temples of Asclepius in Epidaurus, Lebena, and Pergamum) and reflecting deep religious devotion.[47] Pausanias, for example, has a description of the Epidaurian Asclepieion in which 'tablets stood within the enclosure. Of old, there were more of them: in my time six were left. On these tablets are engraved the names of men and women who were healed by Asclepius, together with the disease from which they suffered, and how he was cured. These tablets were written in Doric dialect'.[48] Those writing the tablets were not unaware of a more 'scientific' approach to medicine,

---

[42] Parker (1983) 213.

[43] In the Hippocratic treatise, *Nature of Man*, the author criticized previous philosophers and physicians who held that the human body is constituted by a single element (fire, water, or earth) or by a single humour (blood, bile, or phlegm) before moving into his own explanation of the human body as being constituted by four humours (blood, phegm, yellow bile, and black bile) whose mixture explains health and separations explain disease. Hippoc. *Nat. Hom.* 1–7.

[44] Hippoc. *Nat. Hom.* 8–15.

[45] Cf. Hippoc. *Nat. Hom.* 5 ἢν γάρ τινι διδῷς ἀνθρώπῳ φάρμακον ὅ τι φλέγμα ἄγει, ἐμέεταί σοι φλέγμα, καὶ ἢν διδῷς φάρμακον ὅ τι χολὴν ἄγει, ἐμέεταί σοι χολή. 'If you give a man medicine which withdraws phlegm he will vomit phlegm, if you give him one which withdraws bile he will vomit bile'.

It is noteworthy that this treatise is the only one of the entire Hippocratic corpus to which a known author can be ascribed. It was written by Polybus, Hippocrates' pupil and son-in-law. Jouanna (1999) 400.

[46] Parker (1983) 215.

[47] Chaniotis (1995) 323–324.

[48] στῆλαι δὲ είστήκεσαν ἐντὸς τοῦ περιβόλου τὸ μὲν ἀρχαῖον καὶ πλέονες, ἐπ' ἐμοῦ δὲ ἓξ λοιπαί· ταύταις ἐγγεγραμμένα καὶ ἀνδρῶν καὶ γυναικῶν ἐστιν ὀνόματα ἀκεσθέντων ὑπὸ τοῦ 'Ασκληπιοῦ, προσέτι δὲ καὶ νόσημα ὅ τι ἕκαστος ἐνόσησε καὶ ὅπως ἰάθη· γέγραπται δὲ φωνῇ τῇ Δωρίδι. Paus. 2.27.3. Cf. Str. 8.6.15; Lib. *Ep.* 695.2; Sozom. *Hist. eccl.* 2.5.

as is evident from their reference to prescriptions and methods of healing, but chose a religious approach.[49] A study of the propitiatory inscriptions of Lydia and Phrygia demonstrates just how common was the view that illness was a divine punishment for a sin (usually for a religious offence). Only atonement could therefore provide cure, which proves that illness and sin lay closely together in the Graeco-Roman world.[50] The requirement of Asclepius from his worshippers that they approach him purified in their moral character, which Porphyrius mentioned, and the inscription on the Asclepieion at Lambaeasis, Africa, that a stay in the temple brings moral improvement suggest that the connection between illness and moral impurity and between obtaining cure and moral atonement was widespread.[51]

Nonetheless, a variety of opinions existed on the question of why diseases occurred and what was their nature, and this debate highlighted the issue of the authority and expertise of those suitable to offer care. There were religious men who argued they knew how to appease the gods, but also those of scientific propensity who thought that each disease had a nature and could thus be diagnosed and apprehended with reason, skill, and human knowledge.[52] The duties of the ritual expert stretched from religious ceremonies of pollution and purification to the management of temples to which the sick came to be healed.

To achieve cleansing (*katharsis*) Greek and Roman physicians often used *pharmaka*. However *pharmakon* is not just used in reference to remedies, but also to mean poisons, charms, and spells.[53] Greek and Roman doctors habitually used herbal medicine, which had highly toxic properties and posed an actual threat to the patient's life. The willingness of a patient to follow his physician's instructions was seen as a vote of confidence in the doctor.[54] Such a vote of confidence was imperative for physicians who were,

---

[49] Such a choice did not need to be exclusive and usually it was not.

[50] Chaniotis (1995).

[51] Porphyrius, *De Abstinentia*, 2.19; *CIL* VIII, 1, no. 2584.

[52] Cf. Hippoc. *Morb. Sacr.* 1–3, and *passim*.

[53] Cf. Pl. *Phd.* 57a. See also the stimulating discussions of Artelt (1937) and Derrida (1981). See below, pp. 96–98.

[54] Cf. GOR. μέγα δέ σοι τεκμήριον ἐρῶ· πολλάκις γὰρ ἤδη ἔγωγε μετὰ τοῦ ἀδελφοῦ καὶ μετὰ τῶν ἄλλων ἰατρῶν εἰσελθὼν παρά τινα τῶν καμνόντων οὐχὶ ἐθέλοντα ἢ φάρμακον πιεῖν ἢ τεμεῖν ἢ καῦσαι παρασχεῖν τῷ ἰατρῷ, οὐ δυναμένου τοῦ ἰατροῦ πεῖσαι, ἐγὼ ἔπεισα, οὐκ ἄλλῃ τέχνῃ ἢ τῇ ῥητορικῇ. (And I will give you a strong proof for it. I have often in the past gone with my brother and with other physicians to some sick men not willing to drink drug or to let the physician cut or burn him; when the physician could not persuade him, I persuaded him by no other craft than rhetoric). Pl. *Grg.* 456a–b. This argument of Gorgias demonstrates that being a physician did not guarantee the patient's trust.

setting more speculative issues aside, craftsmen plying their trade.[55] As such, the physician was always in search of patients, and to obtain their patronage he first had to earn their trust. One of the commonest methods of securing this trust was by providing credible prognosis.[56] Indeed, as Ludwig Edelstein demonstrated, by the late fifth and fourth century prognosis was the best way for a physician to establish his reputation.[57] By predicting the future course of his patient's illness to his family and friends the doctor could gain credit for his cure. Even if the patient died, as long as his death was foretold, the physician's reputation stayed intact. In the case of Aristides it is clear that such a vote of confidence was rarely provided, maybe due to his doctors' poor performance.[58]

The importance of prognosis in Hippocratic medicine and its aftermath reveals the influence of traditional forms of prophecy on Greek medicine.[59] Indeed the opening sentence of the Hippocratic treatise *On Prognosis* which advises physicians to practise prognosis 'for if he [i.e. the physician] will discover and declare unaided by the side of his patients the present, the past and the future, and fill in the gaps in the account given by the sick, he will be the more believed to understand the cases, so that men will confidently entrust themselves to him for treatment'.[60] Such a description of the ideal physician with his ability to tell the past, the present and the future bears great resemblance to that of the faculties of the Homeric seers: 'and among them stood up Calchas, the son of Thestor, the best of the bird interpreters, who knew all things that were, the things to be and the things past'.[61] Medical prognosis was taken as the art of knowing the future course of the patient's

---

55 Nutton (2004) 87. The ambiguous social status of physicians in antiquity, either as scientists or as craftsmen, was studied by Horstmanshoff (1990); Deichgräber (1970) looked into the image of physicians in classical antiquity and Pleket (1995) offers a broader view on the social status of physicians in classical antiquity.

56 Hippoc. *Prog.* 1.

57 Edelstein (1937) 65–85; Hippoc. *Prog.* 1.

58 As we shall see, the initial failure of physicians to provide Aristides with an accurate prognosis must have had a long-lasting effect on his relationship with them and limited the trust he placed in them.

59 Jouanna (1999) 100.

60 Τὸν ἰητρὸν δοκέει μοι ἄριστον εἶναι πρόνοιαν ἐπιτηδεύειν· προγιγνώσκων γὰρ καὶ προλέγων παρὰ τοῖσι νοσέουσι τά τε παρεόντα καὶ τὰ προγεγονότα καὶ τὰ μέλλοντα ἔσεσθαι, ὁκόσα τε παραλείπουσιν οἱ ἀσθενέοντες ἐκδιηγεύμενος, πιστεύοιτ' ἂν μᾶλλον γιγνώσκειν τὰ τῶν νοσεόντων πρήγματα, ὥστε τολμᾷν ἐπιτρέπειν τοὺς ἀνθρώπους σφέας ἑωυτοὺς τῷ ἰητρῷ. Hippoc. *Prog.* 1.

61 τοῖσι δ' ἀνέστη / Κάλχας Θεστορίδης οἰωνοπόλων ὄχ' ἄριστος / ὃς ᾔδη τά τ' ἐόντα τά τ' ἐσσόμενα πρό τ' ἐόντα / καὶ νήεσσ' ἡγήσατ' Ἀχαιῶν Ἴλιον εἴσω / ἣν διὰ μαντοσύνην. Hom. *Il.* 1.68–73.

illness from existing signs. Although these signs were not the flight of birds, the entrails of animals or other signs which were traditionally interpreted by soothsayers, the gulf between medical prognosis and that of the priest was narrow enough for the Hippocratic physician and his successors to be confused with magicians when producing accurate prognosis on a regular basis.[62] However, by adopting certain professional traits, such as providing prognosis, it became meaningful to talk about 'knowledge' in the discipline of medicine, as noted by Barton.[63] The sick were taught to expect it, and once given, the healer gained power.

A thorough discussion of the various methods the Hippocratic physician and his successors employed to form a prognosis is outside the scope of this discussion.[64] It is important to note, though, that they all observed signs and symptoms which they assumed to have resulted from the primary causes of these symptoms. In fact, this line of thought was not restricted to practitioners of medicine. Thucydides follows such a pattern in his wide-ranging account of the Athenian plague and his narrative suggests acquaintance with contemporary medical vocabulary.[65] The search for distinctive symptoms in order to form an understanding as to their *cause* (hence forming a notion of disease in a scientific sense and of the human body as a sophisticated machine) thus enabling an accurate diagnosis and prognosis to be formed with the avoidance of mistaken ones, is attestable in the work of Galen.[66] The Hippocratic physician was less concerned with distinguishing between diseases. His prime interest was in the association between certain groups of symptoms and his patient's particular constitution.[67]

It is noteworthy that disease could affect whole groups as well as individuals. The Greek vocabulary to describe disease and health, νοσός and cognates such as νόσημα for disease and ὑγίεια for well-being, has a wider use than the strictly medical.[68] The terminologies used to define what it meant

---

62 The Hippocratic physician spared no effort in his attempts to repudiate the methods of the soothsayers (cf. Hippoc. *Virg.* 1; Hippoc. *Acut.* 8). However, to most people these differences in methodology between medical prognosis and that of the soothsayers must have seemed insignificant, especially having been accustomed to hearing of mythic physicians or physician gods who were also seers, such as Apollo of Delphi (cf. Aesch. *Supp.* 263; *Eum.* 62; *Ag.* 1623).

63 See above, pp. 42–43.

64 See, in addition to Hippoc. *Prog.* discussion in Jouanna (1999) 100–111.

65 Nutton (2004) 22–24, 90.

66 S.W. Jackson (1969) 365–384; Hankinson (1998a) and, more generally (1998b).

67 Hankinson (1981); Nutton (2004) 92.

68 Brock (2000).

to suffer from disease, and what the opposite of being healthy meant, were not restricted to individuals. Groups, cities, and nations could suffer disease. For individual sufferers of disease this could mean 'lack of education', 'madness', or 'senselessness'. For a group it could mean fraction, injustice, tyranny or disorder.[69] In Aeschylus there is disease in tyranny, Demosthenes sees his contemporary Greece 'destroyed by disease'. Herodotus depicts his present day Greeks as healthy in a political sense. Likewise, for Xenophon the whole cosmos is healthy. Thucydides describes ships as healthy. Homer and Plato used *hygieia* to describe a sound mind.[70] The parallels between the human body and the body politic are widespread in Greek literature partly because the Greeks inscribed political and ethical values onto the body and onto nature itself.[71]

A group of people or a political organisation could be described as diseased, and due to a lack of clear paradigmatic guidelines in physiology and medicine it is fair to assume that a distinction between the literal and metaphorical use of medical terms was never drawn in the Graeco-Roman world.[72] As Geoffrey Lloyd explains:

> In diagnoses of why the state is sick, some may concentrate on individuals as pollutants in the body of politics, other on factors of internal strife, (στάσις), and faction constructed on the analogy of the physical diseases that strike the body. The topic of authority, in this context too, is loaded with significance. If you believe the state is diseased, you will need the statesman-doctor to diagnose what is wrong and to prescribe the right cure, dealing with the causes of the problem as pathogens to be excised or purged from the body of politics'.[73]

Aristides himself used this vocabulary in his orations to the Greek cities. The analogy of soul body was commonly used in medical discourse and through it in political discourse regarding matters such as the form of the

---

[69] Lloyd (2003) 12–13.

[70] Aesc. *Pr.* 224–225; X. *Mem.* 4.3.13; Th. 8. 107; Hdt. 7. 157. Hom. *Il.* 8.524; Pl. *R.* 584e; *Tht.* 194b.

[71] The literature on this issue is vast. Cf. Jouanna (1978); (1980a); (1980b); Kallet (1999); Cuomo (2007) 8.

[72] Kuhn defines a paradigm as the achievements of scientists, which at least for a while dominate a particular scientific community (cf. physicians, chemists, biologists etc.), providing both good enough solutions, as well as formulations of related problems. (Kuhn [1962] 9). The existence of a paradigm is paramount for proper science. A paradigm provides models in which science can grow. However, Kuhn also defines a pre-historical stage of a scientific paradigm, in which there are constant arguments as to methodology, criteria, and sufficient proof. (p. 47).

[73] Lloyd (2003) 7.

state and its health (cf. Plato et al.).[74] Diagnosing a social organisation as healthy or diseased was not always done metaphorically, which suggests that the meaning of disease and the understanding of its mechanism were fundamentally different from our own. This notion is explicitly developed in two of Aristides' orations, *Concerning Concord*, and *Panegyric in Cyzicus*.[75] Aristides was no exception: he frequently used medical vocabulary in connection with social and political matters. In the *Roman Oration* Aristides praised Rome for bringing a cure to the entire civilised world by its peaceful government after a long period of sickness.[76] In the context of strife between some of the leading Greek cities in Asia due to a competitive spirit, Aristides delivered speeches in support of concord. Strife, he argued more than once, was a disease of the city.[77] Similarly, when civic disorders occurred in Rhodes Aristides described what should be done in terms of a sick society in need of a doctor.[78] By doing so Aristides joined a long tradition of Greek political thought.

The inability of Graeco-Roman medicine to adopt one coherent and agreed-upon explanatory model or paradigm (scientific, religious or both) to guide all medical activities did not mean that medicine—both as a practice and as a discipline—was in any way hard to define. Medicine, particularly its social aspect, namely the practice of medicine, was well established and recognised. The Greek world was familiar with the professional physician.[79] Medicine in Greek thought was both a discipline and an art (both fall under the Greek term τέχνη).[80] In the dialogues of Plato and the works of Aristotle the image of the physician recurrently appears to embody an artisan who masters the knowledge and practice of medicine. In the *Phaedrus* Plato praised Hippocrates' medical method as the classic model for the dialectical method of the philosopher.[81] In the *Gorgias*, one of the dialogues

74 The earliest example is Solon, 4.17; Thgn. 1133–1134; the lexicographers' terminology also supports this cf. Hesychius has *nosos*: *stasiazon* and Pollux 8.152, ascribes a similar sense to *nosos*. See also Dem. 2.14; 9.12; Ar. *Vesp*. 650–651 demonstrates that this use of the term *nosos* in a social and political contexts was common enough to have been used in parody. Brock (2000) 33.

75 See here the illuminating discussion of Petsalis-Diomidis (2008).

76 Aristid. *Or*. 26. 97–98K.

77 E.g. Aristid. *Or*. 24. 16, 18, 31 K.

78 Aristid. *Or*. 24 K.

79 For epigraphical evidence Cf. Samama (2003).

80 This view dates back to the beginning of the sixth century BC: Stob. 3.9.23 = Solon, *Fr*. 13. 41–52 W. For a study of the meaning of the Greek term τέχνη see Cuomo (2007) 7–40.

81 Pl. *Phdr*. 270c–d.

of Plato's first period, the Platonic Socrates pronounces his advance of a new kind of philosophy, the object of which is the care of the soul. This new philosophy aims to follow the model of the art of the physician, whose task is to care for the human body, and he [i.e. Plato's Socrates] determines its scientific character by deriving from this medical model the constitutive elements of a true art (τέχνη).[82] Aristotle later adopted this philosophical method in his *Nicomachean Ethics*.[83] The clear voice of Plato and Aristotle, amongst other classical Greek authors in regards to medicine as a discipline and as a profession later played a seminal role in shaping the conceptual scheme of Aristides and other *pepaideumenoi*, who continuously harked back to this golden age of Greek culture in quest of their own identity.

Although medicine was perceived as a discipline and physicians formed a group of professionals, the practice and study of medicine in classical antiquity was much less canonised than it may first appear. This situation is illustrated in respect of the existence and use of professional jargon and vocabulary. Names of specific diseases, which can lead to the erroneous conclusion that there was a canonised system of nosology, were, in fact, used in a very loose manner. The term φθίσις, to take but one example, which we usually translate as tuberculosis, could cover a variety of other wasting diseases.[84] Sores, gangrenes and abscesses were all seen as one disease. Furthermore, there was no way of guaranteeing that one physician's terminology agreed with that of another. Galen's critique of 'younger physicians' who introduced new typologies is indicative of a common habit rather than being a first step towards a solution.[85]

Most of the literary evidence for ancient medical practice is preserved either in the Hippocratic corpus or in the work of Galen.[86] From the earliest times, however, therapies might involve incantation (e.g. to staunch the flood of blood from a wound sustained from fighting a wild boar: *Od.* 19. 452–458), or the use of analgesic drugs (by Patroclus, for example: *Il.* 11. 837–848), or the magical herb *moly* to defend Odysseus against Circe's witchcraft (*Od.* 10. 203–347), down to the use of amulets and charms by the so-called 'purifiers' and 'magicians'. Medical treatment was also provided by drug-sellers, midwives, root-cutters, gymnastic trainers, and surgeons.

---

82 Pl. *Grg.* 464 sq. 500e sq. Jaeger (1957) 54.
83 Jaeger (1957) 54.
84 Nutton (2004) 28; Grmek (1989) 177–197.
85 Nutton (2004) 28–29; Gal. *On Medical Terminology*.
86 It is noteworthy that the Hippocratic Corpus and the work of Galen stood more than five centuries apart from one another.

The history of Greek medicine is interwoven with the history of Greek religion. In a study of Aristides, particular attention must be drawn to the history of the cult of Asclepius and to the history of Asclepius' temples and their function as medical centres. In classical Greece, which Aristides, like other *pepaideumenoi* saw as the ultimate point of reference, shrines and temples to the god Asclepius formed one important focus for religious medicine.[87] The cult of Asclepius was initially introduced in Athens after the great plague but the spread of the cult of Asclepius did not stop in Athens.[88] By the middle of the fourth century BCE the cult of Asclepius and his family members Hygieia, Panacea and Epione had spread all over the Greek-speaking world. The cult was practised from Cyrene on the coast of Africa to the island of Thasos in the north Aegean and from Asia Minor to Sicily.[89] Associations of Asclepius' worshippers are attested to from the fourth century BCE well into late antiquity. Both the spread of the cult of Asclepius and its perseverance are remarkable.[90] It is interesting to note that Hippocratic medicine developed in fifth century Athens and the Aegean at the very same time that Asclepius turned from a hero into a god.[91] Already in the fifth and fourth centuries BCE shrine medicine was common in the Greek world and by far the most important medical centres associated with Asclepius or any other deity were in Epidaurus and Cos.[92] Archaeology, epigraphy, and later items of literary evidence depict the nature of help and advice one was likely to receive there.[93] A range of problems were addressed in the Asclepieia, but most were of a medical nature.[94]

[87] Ancient testimony relating to the cult of Asclepius is collected in E. Edelstein and L. Edelstein Vol. i. (1945).

[88] For the arrival of the cult of Asclepius to Athens during the Eleusinian Mysteries in 420 BCE see *SIG* 88. Tradition has it that Sophocles made his own house a place of worship to the god until a temple was built (cf. Plut. *Num.* 3; *TrGF* 4 T69). Moreover, an Athenian inscription from the third century CE records the opening of Sophocles' famous paean to Asclepius. For the inscription itself see *SEG* XXVIII 225; *IG* III I (1978), addenda p. 490 n. 171; Furley and Bremer vol. ii (2001) 219–221. Ancient references to Sophocles' paean are: Lucian, *Encom. Demosth.* 27; Philostr. *VA* 3.17 = *TrGF* 4T 73a.

[89] Edelstein & Edelstein vol. i (1945) T 716–799.

[90] Nutton (2004) 106.

[91] Krug (1985) 120–187. But cf. Gorrini (2005) for a compeling explanation for the intrinsic connections between temple medicine and Hippocratic medicine.

[92] Krug (1985)128–134.

[93] Most evidence is collected by E. and L. Edelstein (1945) T. 382–553. See also van Straten (1981) for the archaeological evidence.

[94] E.g. treatment of a festering wound: *Anth. Pal.* 6.330; eye problems: Ael. *Fragmenta*, 100; gout, fever and headaches: Epict. *Dissertationes*, 4.8.28–29.

This close affinity between medicine, magic, and religion lasted throughout antiquity and beyond.[95]

The intrinsic connection between medicine and religion was not restricted to the temple. An archaeological study (in a Foucaultian sense) of medical knowledge in antiquity and its phenomenology (the way that things—objects, images, ideas, emotions—appear or are present in consciousness) reveals much common ground between medical and religious thought.[96] In the case of Aristides this common ground comes into play most vigorously when we turn to his appeals to and reliance on Asclepius and, more concretely, to the function of dreams in his treatment. As we shall see, Aristides' understanding of the dream mechanism, the role of the gods in sending dreams, and the place such views had in the Graeco-Roman health-care system, resembles that of other Graeco-Roman philosophers, doxographers and physicians. Furthermore, none of these notions was an invention of Aristides, nor was he responsible for positioning them in the Graeco-Roman health-care system.

Graeco-Roman medical knowledge is itself an area which lies between opinion and scientific facts (in a modern sense), and is embodied not only in theoretical texts or experimental instruments, but in a whole body of practices and institutions. Foucault's *Birth of the Clinic* and *Archaeology of Knowledge* allow us to see that medicine is not simply a mechanical practice, but also a language which has evolved over time. Foucault's notion of archaeology, which means the uncovering of the grid of knowledge which organises every scientific discourse and defines what can and what cannot be thought scientifically, is paramount to a proper understanding of Aristides' experiences as a sick person. Medical discourses in general organise themselves in relation to certain structures—political, social, cultural and economic—and to each other.[97] A particular arrangement of a medical discourse affects the way things are seen and are spoken of and draws the borderline between what belongs to the medical discourse and what does not. Medicine simply reorganises illness as a disease according to a new pattern of syntax. Our perception of the body as the natural space of the origin and distribution of disease, a space determined by the anatomical atlas, is merely one of the various ways in which medicine forms its knowledge.[98]

---

95 Lloyd (1979); Lloyd (1982); Lloyd (1991).
96 Cf. Bates (1995); Amundsen (1996); Grmek (1998).
97 Cf. Good (1994).
98 Horrocks and Jevtic (1997) 55.

The absence of a medical paradigm (in its modern sense) or even an agreement on the proper context in which to place medical discourse in Aristides' day and culture is vividly demonstrated by a dinner table debate (either real or imagined) in a work of Plutarch concerning the appearance of new types of diseases, a common theme in the first century CE.[99] The first speaker, a local physician, argued in favour of the possibility of the appearance of new types of disease, supporting his claim by a quote of a treatise of Athenodorus on epidemics (both author and work are otherwise unknown). This Athenodorus argued that rabies and 'elephantiasis' were not familiar before the age of Asclepiades. Diogenianus, the next speaker, strongly objects. His argument was that the whole notion of atoms coming from outside the universe and bringing new types of disease, an argument which rested at the foundation of the Democritean and possibly Asclepiadean schools, is wrong. For Diogenianus all types of disease are caused by specific dietary habits and, therefore, form a finite set. Plutarch himself has the last word. He accepted the possibility of new types of disease, but rejected them coming from outside the universe. New diseases, Plutarch explained, must have simple causes.

Medical discourse, it appears from Plutarch's dinner talk, was inherently connected to the fields of philosophy of nature, cosmology and ultimately theology and religion. When Plutarch and his guests were making a judgement about medicine, such as addressing the nature of disease or the constitution of the body, they were expected to make a broader argument about the nature of the world. This type of argument was often indistinguishable from theology. It is within this conceptual scheme that Aristides' experience of being ill and seeking medical help must be set.

Roman Medicine and Its Greek Influences

The adaptation of Greek medicine by the Latin-speaking world is one of the most important moments in the history of medicine.[100] The Roman world appropriated Greek medicine, alongside its explanatory models and professional vocabulary. Roman authors translated Greek medical terminology into Latin, without which medical practice is impossible, by transliterating, translating to an existing Latin equivalent or merely coining Latin

99 Plut. *Table Talks* 8.9 = *Mor.* 731b–734d. For Plutarch and medicine in general see Boulogne (1996).

100 Nutton (2004) 157.

words which kept their original Greek meanings.[101] In turn, Roman authors imported into the Latin speaking world the Greek modes of thinking regarding ailment and health care.[102] The works of philologists demonstrate how it was common to use medical terms of Greek origin, in third century BCE Rome.[103] Even Cato, a fierce opponent of the influence of Greek culture on Roman society, uses a wide range of medical notions of Greek descent in his treatise *On Agriculture*.

It is impossible to talk about the assimilation of Greek medicine in Rome without mentioning Asclepiades of Bithynia.[104] Tradition has it that Asclepiades migrated to Rome where he enjoyed an unsurpassed reputation due to his exceptional cures.[105] The less supportive commentator, Pliny the Elder, noted that Asclepiades became a physician only after he failed in his first career choice, that of a teacher of rhetoric.[106] Nevertheless, there is no doubt that Asclepiades made a significant impression in Rome and that his medical theories and practices were enduring. Their long-term effects were accentuated by the fact that prospective students came from all over the Roman world to study under Asclepiades' supervision in Rome.[107]

The first Roman works which were dedicated either solely or partially to medicine and have survived are Cornelius Celsus' *De Medicina*, and Pliny the Elder's *Historia Naturalis*. Celsus composed an encyclopaedia of which the surviving eight books tell the history of Greek medicine and discuss the origin of dietetics and of medical theory (book 1 with proem), pathology and therapeutics (book 2), special treatments (book 3–4), drug-lore (book 5–6), surgery (book 7), and skeletal anatomy (book 8).[108] The importance of Celsus' work here is twofold: as a source for the history of Greek medicine

---

101 Ibid.

102 The ability of language to share the comprehension of reality is one of the central conclusions of Kleinman, Geertz, Wittgenstein, and Hablwachs; see pp. 3, 40–44.

103 Cf. the medical jokes of Plautus; Langslow (1999) 183–226.

104 Rawson (1982) 358 claimed that 'it can be argued that there was no intellectual figure at work in Rome in the period of the late Republic who had more originality and influence than the Bithynian doctor Asclepiades'. The chronology of Asclepiades' life and arrival in Rome are still not beyond dispute. For accounts of Asclepiades' life see Rawson (1982) and Polito (1999).

105 Apuleius, *Anthology*, 4.19.

106 Plin. *Nat. Hist.* 7.37.124.

107 Nutton (2004) 168.

108 The prooemium to book 1 is one of the most important ancient sources for the history of medicine, covering the period from the Homeric epics to Celsus' own day. Valuable discussions of Celsus' Prooemium are: Deuse (1993) and the notes in the edition of Mudry (1982).

and as evidence for the familiarity of Greek medicine in the Roman world of the first century CE.[109] Pliny's *Historia Naturalis* is a thirty-seven book encyclopaedia of all contemporary knowledge.[110]

Both works encapsulate the Roman attitude towards the art of medicine in the first century CE. Neither author was a professional physician, but they were upper class Romans of an inquisitive nature. They were wealthy landowners who embodied the Roman ideal of the self-sufficient *paterfamilias*, a man of wide learning and practical outlook. They regarded part of medicine as a craft, which they thought they had mastered by reading and experience. Neither saw a compelling need for formal medical studies. A professional physician was not a part of the *mos maiorum*.[111] Pliny advised his reader to consider a doctor's advice with the utmost care. Only a physician, he commented, could kill without being punished: 'I shall not even attempt to denounce their avarice, the rapacious haggling while their patients' fate hangs in the balance'.[112]

However, Aristides' comprehension of medicine and its interrelationship with religion, particularly the cult of Asclepius, were not alien to the Romans.[113] Celsus writes in the prooemium to his *De Medicina*:

> *Ut alimenta sanis corporibus agricultura, sic sanitatem aegris medicina promittit. Haec nusquam quidem non est, siquidem etiam inperitissimae gentes herbas aliaque promta in auxilium vulnerum morborumque noverunt. Verum tamen apud Graecos aliquanto magis quam in ceteris nationibus exculta est, ac ne apud hos quidem a prima origine, sed paucis ante nos saeculis. Ut pote cum vetustissimus auctor Aesculapius celebretur, qui quoniam adhuc rudem et vulgarem hanc scientiam paulo subtilius excoluit, in deorum numerum receptus est. Huius deinde duo filii Podalirius et Machaon bello Troiano ducem Agamemnonem secuti non mediocrem opem commilitonibus suis attulerunt.*[114]
>
> Just as agriculture promises nourishment to healthy bodies, so does the art of medicine promise health to the sick. Nowhere is this art wanting, for even the most uncivilised nations have had the knowledge of herbs, and

---

[109] For the role of Celsus in translating Greek medical terminology into Latin see Langslow (1994).

[110] Pliny's work is unrivalled is terms of scale of the works to have reached us from classical antiquity. Nicholas Purcell has commented that the study of medicine (alongside other aspects of the classical world) would have been substantially impoverished without Pliny's work. Purcell (1996).

[111] Jackson (1988) 10.

[112] *'Ne avaritiam quidem arguam rapacesque nundias pendentibus fatis'*. Plin. *Nat. Hist.* 29. 8. 18–21. For Pliny's general attitude towards Greek physicians see Hahn (1991).

[113] The cult of Asclepius was first introduced in Rome by the early 3rd century BC and in 293 BC a temple was dedicated to Asclepius on the *Insula Tiberina*.

[114] Cels. *Prooem.* 1–3.

other things to hand for aiding of wounds and diseases. This art, however, has been cultivated among the Greeks much more than in other nations—not, however, even among them from their first beginnings, but only for a few generations before ours. Hence Asclepius is celebrated as the most ancient authority, and because he cultivated this science, as yet rude and vulgar, with a little more than common refinement, he was numbered among the gods. After him his two sons, Podaleirius and Machaon, who followed Agamemnon as the leader to the Trojan War, gave not inconsiderable help to their comrades.

According to Celsus, medicine as a discipline evolved only after literary studies began: *Primoque medendi scientia sapientiae pars habebatur, ut et morborum curatio et rerum naturae contemplatio sub isdem auctoribus nata sit*[115] (At first the science of healing was held to be part of philosophy, so that treatment of disease and contemplation on the nature of things began through the same authorities). Celsus' narrative is imbued with Roman tradition. He argues that literary life benefits the mind but disagrees with the body, which is why:

> *Scilicet is hanc maxime requirentibus, qui corporum suorum robora quieta cogitatione nocturnaque vigilia minuerant. Ideoque multos ex sapientiae professoribus peritos eius fuisse accipimus, clarissimos vero ex is Pythagoran et Enpedoclen et Democritum.*[116]

> Healing was needed especially by those whose bodily strength was weakened by restless thinking and night-watching. Hence we find that many who professed philosophy became experts in medicine, the most celebrated being Pythagoras, Empedocles, and Democritus.

Celsus also provides evidence for the evolution of Greek medicine and for its dependence on philosophy. The first physician to have drawn a distinction between medicine and philosophy, according to Celsus, was Hippocrates of Cos.[117]

It would be mistaken, however, to depict the role of Rome in a history of ancient medicine as merely reactive to Greek views. Of the three schools of classical-age medicine—Rationalism, Empiricism, and Methodism—the rise of Methodism in the first century CE is the single most important Roman

115 Cels. *Prooem.* 6. Other authors of the Roman era, such Galen, and the author of Ps. Galen *Introductio sive medicus* 14.674–797K were equally incline to see Asclepius as the founder of Hippocratic medicine. Cf. Petit (2010) 343–347.

116 Cels. *Prooem.* 7–8.

117 Cels. *Prooem.* 8.

contribution to medicine.[118] Methodism was motivated by dissatisfaction with both Empiricist and Hippocratic approaches to diagnosis.[119] It offered a new epistemology of medicine as an ongoing process of knowledge based on a correlation between observation and a small range of underlying conditions. As the name of this school suggests, the presupposition of Methodism was the possibility of formulating and following a successful method of healing. This school dominated medical theory throughout the Roman world for at least three centuries.[120] Galen's rival as an imperial physician in 170s Rome, Statilius Attalus, was a Methodist who descended from the same Asia Minor family as Statilius Crito.[121] Furthermore, unlike the works of rationalist and empiricist physicians, who wrote solely in Greek, Methodism was bilingual. A treatise from the North African physician Caelius Aurelianus on *Chronic and Acute Diseases* was composed in Latin. Soranus of Ephesus, on the other hand, also a renowned Methodist of the second century, wrote his work on *Gynaecology* in Greek.

According to Celsus and Pliny it was Themison who laid the ground work for Methodism. He had argued that good medicine was simply effective practice. Themison saw no need for complex systems of nosology and nosological classifications to search for a disease's hidden causes, but he did not dismiss nosology and observation altogether.[122] However, empirical observation by itself was not enough. The Methodists argued that all diseases shared some general and visible attributes, which they described as a search for 'common features' (κοινότης). Once these 'commonalities' were properly identified, a suitable treatment could be offered. An investigation into the origin of these commonalities—a common quest amongst Hippocratic physicians—was not the physician's task and, in any case, irrelevant for the choice of treatment. Likewise, an attempt to find precedents in past cases, as the Empiricists instructed, was time consuming, and, in the absence of any particular principle to direct this sort of a search, futile.[123]

A later Methodist, Thessalus, turned the 'commonalities' into the central notion of Methodism.[124] These commonalities became increasingly subdivided: firstly between those concerning dietetic habits and those con-

---

118 For a history of Methodism see Frede (1982), Rubinstein (1985) and Gourevitch (1991).
119 Nutton (2004) 187–188.
120 Celsus, *Med.* prooem. 53.
121 Gal. 10.909–916 K; for Crito see Nutton (2004) 256.
122 Celsus, *Med.* prooem. 64.
123 Nutton (2004) 191.
124 Gal. 18.271, 10.35 K.

cerning surgery; then the surgical commonalities themselves had a number of sub-categories.[125] Once the indicators of a certain commonality were detected, the treatment had to follow a rigid and predetermined path.

The fundamental disagreement between Methodists and between Galen and the Hippocratic tradition was in their approach to the issue of acquisition of medical knowledge. Galen, like the Hippocratics, perceived medicine as a science, which meant there was a coherent system of data and also principles of drawing conclusions from this data. The Methodists, on the other hand, saw medical practice as an attempt to understand, rather than identify, a certain state of affairs within a pre-composed body of evidence.[126]

It was not simply medical knowledge that the Roman world appropriated from the Greek. In 423 BCE, historians claim, the Greek deity of Apollo the Healer had been introduced in Rome to help battle an epidemic. A century and a half later an even more dramatic event occurred. In 293 BCE, after three years of deadly epidemic in Rome, Roman priests consulted the Sibylline Books and were advised to summon Asclepius to the city. In the following year an official embassy, headed by Quintus Ogulnius, was sent by the Roman senate to invite the god from Epidaurus. Asclepius accepted the Roman invitation and, in the form of a snake, was brought back to Rome. Valerius Maximus tells us that the snake himself chose Tiber Island as his place of residence. A temple was duly dedicated there. The plague soon stopped 'with miraculous speed' (*mira celeritate*) and Asclepius was credited.[127] Rome's acquaintance, it appears, with Greek temple medicine in general and with the cult of Asclepius in particular can be traced back to the early third BC with certainty, and possibly as far back as the fifth century BCE, even before the arrival in Rome of Greek medical works.

The arrival of Greek medicine and Greek physicians in Rome is attributable to two factors: urbanisation and the Hellenisation of Italian culture.[128] By the middle of the first century BCE it was commonplace in high Roman circles to employ a Greek physician. For instance Artemidorus, a Greek physician who was granted Roman citizenship in 80 BCE by C. Cornelius

125 Gal. 1.82 K.

126 Gourevitch (1991) 64–66 citing Gal. *Medical Definitions*, 16–17: 19, 353.

127 Val. Max. is the most detailed account, but certain details are added by Ov. *Met.* 15.622, and the anonymous author of *De Viris Illustribus*, 22.1–3. Valerius depends heavily on Livy, but unfortunately his eleventh book now exists only in an abridgement. It is also possible that Valerius drew information from Varro's *Religious Antiquities*. See p. 58, n. 113 above.

128 Nutton (2004) 163.

Dolabella, was later associated with the circle of Verres.[129] Cicero recommended another Greek physician, one Asclapo of Patras, to his friend Sulpicius Rufus.[130]

In 46 BCE Julius Caesar granted citizenship to all foreign doctors working in Rome. At about the same time in the city of Ephesus doctors were honoured with tax immunity.[131] In 23 BCE or shortly afterwards Augustus is said to have honoured his Greek physician Antonius Musa, who was responsible for the Princeps' miraculous cure, by granting tax immunities to all those who practised medicine.[132] This policy continued during the high empire.[133] Immunities from certain municipal liturgies and tax benefits were bestowed upon physicians, alongside rhetors, philosophers, and grammarians by successive Roman emperors throughout the second century CE.[134] All of these examples demonstrate the high prestige of the medical profession, whose members were mostly of Greek descent.[135] The number of immigrant doctors who seized this opportunity and migrated to Rome hoping to capitalise on its prosperous economy and to secure Roman citizenship is unknown. However, it is certain that medicine maintained an enduring image as being something Greek, which meant that however prosperous and dignified a physician might be, medicine was not deemed a suitable career choice for a proper Roman.[136]

Galen

Galen of Pergamum is a pivotal figure in the history of medicine and his importance exceeds the sphere of medical innovation *per se*. Galen's work redefined the scope of medical discourse and medical practice, and he maintained this pre-eminent status for over a millennium.[137] Galen's views

---

[129] Cic. ii *Verr.* 3.28.

[130] Cic. *Fam.* 13.20.

[131] Suet. *Jul.* 42; *I.Eph.* 4101; Knibbe (1981–1982) 136–140. For the public physicians of ancient Greece see Cohn-Haft (1956).

[132] Suet. *Aug.* 59; Cass. Dio 53.30.

[133] Cf. *IG* IX 1, 104; *I. Delphes*, 462 = *SGDI*, 2632; *SEG* 13 (1956) 361; Cohn-Haft (1956), no. 64; *I. Cret.* I ch. 22, no. 4 p. 245 sqq.

[134] Bowersock (1969) 30–42. A note of the Severan jurist Herrenius Modestinus, in his *Liber Secundus Excusationum* proves that these immunities were not curtailed by Antoninus Pius and his successors, as Bowersock suggested; cf. Dig. 27. 1. 6. 10 with Nutton (1971a) 52, and *passim*.

[135] Jackson (1988) 56.

[136] Nutton (2004) 165.

[137] Nutton (2004) 216; Roy Porter, the social historian of medicine, dedicates no less than eight pages in his history of medicine. Porter (1998) 73–80.

of medicine and medical care are of particular importance for a history of Aristides' malady, both because Galen's work encompassed a description and analysis of much of the medical knowledge and practices up to his own day, including those he discredited, and because of the more general relevance of his work to a social and cultural history of the Graeco-Roman world.[138] Moreover, Galen's choice to present himself as having been encouraged to study medicine by a dream Asclepius sent to his father Nicon is especially meaningful in a study which aims to contextualise the experiences of Aelius Aristides in his present day field of medicine.[139] Marking Asclepius as the instigator of his medical career and a dream as the medium in which this massage was conveyed to Galen's father is consistent with Galen's life-long habit of displaying reverence towards the god of medicine and accepting the possibility of dream as a means of communication between Asclepius and his worshippers.[140]

Being a student in Pergamum at the same time that Aristides convalesced in the Pergamene Asclepieion,[141] and sharing at least two mutual acquaintances with Aristides, Galen's testimony has particular relevance to a study of the *Sacred Tales*. The first of these mutual acquaintances was the physician Satyrus who was Galen's teacher and Aristides' doctor.[142] The second was none other than the Pergamene proconsular L. Cuspius Pactumeius Rufinus, the builder of the exquisite new temple of Zeus-Asclepius in Pergamum, who was an intimate of Aristides and who is also mentioned by Galen.[143] Glen Bowersock, who was mainly interested in Galen's activities as an erudite intellectual and his part in the social and cultural phenomenon known as 'Second Sophistic', thought that 'the fact that he [i.e. Galen] was in Pergamum at the same time as Aristides and had at least two acquaintances

138 Cf. Bowersock (1969) 57–75; Nutton (2004) 230–247.

139 Gal. *Ord. Lib. Prop.* 19. 59 = *SM* 2. 88. 13–17.

140 Asclepius as the father of medicine: Gal. *Protrepticus*, 9. 22; accepting the story of a patient with whom Asclepius communicated via dreams and then treating him: Gal. *Subfiguratio Empirica*, Cp. 10, p. 78 (ed. Deichgräber); expressing reverence towards Asclepius: Gal. *Lib. Prop.* 2. Furthermore, during the Germanic Wars of Marcus Aurelius Galen politely declined an imperial request to join the campaign, claiming Asclepius forbade him to do so: Gal. *Lib. Prop.* 19. 18–19 = *SM* 2. 99. 6–13. Elsewhere Galen records having been directed to therapies by divine dream injunction, cf. Gal. *Cur. Rat. Ven. Sect.* 11. 314–315; *MM* 10. 971–972. An excellent study of Galen's rhetoric of healing is Mattern (2008).

141 Bowersock (1969) 61. On Galen's career cf. Hankinson (2007) 1–33.

142 Gal. 2.224; 19.58 K.

143 Aristid. *Or.* 50.83–84, 107 K; *PIR*^{2}, C 1637. For the Pergamene Asclepieion see Habicht (1969); Hoffmann (1998); Radt (1988); Petsalis-Diomiidis (2010) 151–279, and *passim*.

in common would be enough to prompt speculation that he met the great sophist himself, only twelve years his senior'.[144]

The glory and fame of Galen epitomised the high repute of medicine in general and of Greek physicians in particular in Aristides' world: Galen was born in Pergamum in 129 CE,[145] his father, Nicon, was an educated man, mainly in the field of geometry and architecture, and the young Galen obtained the finest philosophical, literary, and scientific education of his age.[146] Galen was encouraged to study medicine by a dream Asclepius sent to his father Nicon.[147] When his father died Galen left Pergamum to further his studies in Smyrna, Corinth, and Alexandria and did not return to Pergamum for over a decade. We know little of Galen's studies (under Aeschrion, Satyrus, Stratonicus, and Aeficianus in Pergamum, under Pelops and Philippus at Smyrna, and with a variety of teachers in Alexandria), save that they were all described as Hippocratic and displayed a concern with anatomy.[148] Nutton argues that 'the significance of Galen's education cannot be overestimated, since it established, to his ever-repeated satisfaction, the basic principles of proper medicine as he understood it'.[149] It remains to be seen whether Aristides' perception of medicine resembled those of the physician Galen.

Galen's education was, however, exceptional in its length and academic intensity. His library was exceptionally large and he himself was remarkably prolific.[150] Galen's advice to a potential patient seeking a physician was to interview prospective candidates and examine their knowledge of the theories of the great physicians of the past.[151] He may have aimed for a career as a sophist with a medical education, rather than as a practising doctor. The fact that some physicians shared a similar social status to other intellectuals supports such a hypothesis. The prestige of physicians in Galen's world is attested by an inscription from Ephesus which associated physicians,

---

144 Bowersock (1969) 61. It is, however, noteworthy that Bowersock provides no proof for such an encounter. His argument, though highly plausible, is circumstantial.

145 Such definitive dating is possible from Gal. 15.599–600 K.

146 Swain (1996) 357; Nutton (2004) 216–229.

147 Gal. 10. 608 K; 14.608: *CMG* 5.8.1.78 (pl.); 16.223; 19.59 K. Trans. Singer (1997) 27; Nutton (2004) 217.

148 Nutton (2004) 217.

149 Nutton (2004) 218.

150 Nutton (2004) 218–219.

151 Gal. *On Examining a Physician, CMG* Suppl. Or. 4 *passim*. Galen's presupposition was, of course, that the patient himself had profound acquaintance with these works.

alongside sophists, with the city's museum.[152] Another Ephesian inscription makes the connection between physicians and the museum even more explicit.[153] Similarly, in matters of tax-exemptions, physicians and sophists shared an equal status, not just in Ephesus.[154] Galen himself was educated enough to compete with the sophists by mastering Attic Greek and mustering the classical authorities to support his arguments and defeat the sophists at their own game.[155] His acquaintance with the Hippocratic Corpus was remarkable and his use of Plato to prove the logical qualities of the Hippocratic Corpus employed all the authority Greek scholarship could offer.[156]

Galen's other main intellectual influence was philosophy.[157] In this respect he resembled his contemporaries, the Sceptic Sextus Empiricus and the physician Heraclitus of Rhodiapolis.[158] Galen's philosophy and his medicine interacted throughout his life and he strove for a unified art of medicine in which the effective treatment of a patient rested on a thorough understanding of the body alongside an intimate acquaintance with all types of therapy.[159] The opening books of the *Method of Healing* are an exercise in applying logic to the basic notions of medicine and his diagnostics manifest accurate arguments. In turn his discoveries provide support for both Aristotle's notion of a purposeful creator in his *On the Use of Parts of the Body* and for Plato's tripartite bodily system in *On the Opinions of Hippocrates and Plato*. Galen's book on causation, a central topic for Stoics,[160] is an important contribution both to the philosophical discourse and to the practice of doctors.[161] Galen argued that erudition was pertinent to medical knowledge,

---

152 I.*Eph*. 3239. For memberships of physicians in the museums of some of the leading cities of the Graeco-Roman world in the second century, Nutton (1971b) is essential; Millar (1977) 505–506 looks into the association of physicians (alongside philosophers, grammarians and rhetors) to civic museums in his discussion of the Roman government and emperor; Trapp (2007) discusses the association of scholars to cities' museums, in the context of philosophy, scholarship and the world of learning under the Severans.

153 *I.Eph*. 4101 A is a record of a decree of the *boule* and the *demos* concerning *iatroi* 117/31 AD.

154 *Dig*. 50.4.18.30.

155 For the relations between Galen and the so-called second sophistic see Kollesch (1981).

156 Nutton (2004) 218.

157 On Galen's philosophical views see Hankinson (1992).

158 Nutton (2004) 221. Heraclitus of Rhodiapolis was a priest of Asclepius and Hygieia and erected a temple in their honour. Not much is known about him and we have to infer most details from inscriptions. Cf. *TAM* 2.2.910 = *IGRR* 3.733.

159 Nutton (2004) 230.

160 Cf. Sandbach (1975) 81–82, 102, 131.

161 Nutton (2004) 223.

and therefore to medical practice, because it is the only way to be intimately acquainted with the Hippocratic Corpus, which, for Galen, was the supreme medical authority.[162]

Galen's influence was not restricted to the Greek world. In the summer of 162 CE he left Pergamum for Rome where he made a name for himself by public anatomical displays and by his connections with famous patients and friends. His first patient in Rome was his old philosophy teacher, Eudemus. Eudemus enabled Galen to enter the imperial court where he immediately made contacts with the likes of the consul Sergius Paulus and Flavius Boethus, members of the imperial family and other leading figures.[163] Life in Rome, particularly with the fear of the spreading plague, did not agree with Galen and he returned to Pergamum in the summer of 166 CE.[164] Galen was later summoned to join Marcus Aurelius in his campaign against the German tribes, which led him back to Rome during 168 CE. Unfortunately for both Galen and the emperor, Asclepius forbade Galen in a dream to join the emperor in his German campaign. This Asclepian interdiction forced even Marcus Aurelius to yield.[165] However, from this point onwards until the end of his life Galen stayed mainly in Rome.

Galen's views on the proper practice of medicine cannot be easily summarised. Information has to be derived from his many works, some of which are directed to patients, some to physicians and yet others to students of medicine. The one area which unites them is Galen's insistence on his ability to teach medicine, in its true and Hippocratic sense, because he was both a scholar and a practitioner. In fact, Galen believed was that one cannot claim authority in medical matters simply by having read the appropriate literature; experience is crucial. In this respect Galen was much closer to the Empiricists, with their acquired experimental knowledge, than to those who compiled medical works based on theory alone.[166] However, Galen insisted on the importance of theoretical knowledge alongside praxis and on the requirement for profound acquaintance with the human anatomy.[167] In order to gain such knowledge he viewed dissection as indispensible and

---

[162] Nutton (2004) 219–221.

[163] Nutton (2004) 224.

[164] The air of anxiety in the streets of Rome on the eve of Marcus' German campaign is vividly captured in the pages of Lucian, *Alex.* 48 ff.

[165] Gal. 19.18 K; trans. Singer (1997) 7–8; 14.4; trans. Brock (1929) 197; 14.650; *CMG* 5, 8, 1, 118–121. Nutton (2004) 225.

[166] Frede (1981) 65–86.

[167] Galen, 2.225, 343, 643–646 K: trans. Singer (1956) 5, 61, 197–199; *On the Examining Physician* 9.23; 14.1–4: *CMG* Suppl. Or. 4.114–115, 134–137; Nutton (2004) 230.

vivisection as useful. Indeed, Galen explains how to perform such a procedure in depth in his *Anatomical Procedures* and in two other works (which we now know only from their Arabic translation) on dissection and vivisection.[168] Galen's anatomical explorations confirmed the wisdom and foresight of god, or the *Creator of Nature* (ὁ δημιουργός),[169] as Galen refers to him interchangeably.[170] Each one of nature's creations—the eye of an insect, the trunk of the elephant or the human hand—was perfectly designed.[171]

Galen's intimate acquaintance with human anatomy made him a successful physician. He was able to restore sensation in the hand of the Syrian sophist Pausanias who suffered a riding accident because he was familiar with the inner structure of the hand's nervous system.[172] Galen also emphasised the interrelations between mind and body, and particularly the physical hazards of mental stress.[173] Such an understanding of mind-body relations shaped Galen's perception of the role of the physician. Like Aristotle before him, Galen saw a continuum between the role of the physician and that of the philosopher, and Galen claimed jurisdiction over issues of morality as well. Nutton explains: 'It was not enough for the doctor to act as the candid friend and to point out the consequences that might ensue from the passions and errors of the soul—a task for which Galen considered himself well qualified from his daily reading and rereading of the so-called *Golden Words* of Pythagoras. He could now offer medical advice that would remove or mitigate them and restore moral as well as physical well-being'.[174] In this capacity, the role of the physician was not far removed from that of the priest.

---

168 Nutton (2004) 231.

169 Gal. *De usu partium*. 11.14 = 3. 905 K = p. 158 Helmreich.

170 Galen's thoughts about theology exceed my scope here. However, as Frede demonstrated [Frede (2003) 84], Galen not only had a detailed theological position, he also found it relevant to medicine [Gal. *PHP* 7, 9, 12, p. 588, 20–22 De Lacy = V 780, 16–17 K]. In another comment in a treatise on the use of parts [*UP* II pp. 447, 22–448, 3 Helmreich = IV 360, 15–361, 1 K] Galen argued that the use of the parts is useful not merely to the physician, but also to the philosopher who pursues a comprehensive knowledge of nature. Here, Frede explains, Galen thinks of theology as a philosophical discipline 'a discipline one will pursue if one tries to understand the whole of nature' [Frede (2003) 85]. This is anything but revolutionary. After all, the followers of Plato, Aristotle, and the Stoics perceived god as a principle of nature.

171 Hankinson (1989) 206–227; also relevant here is Jouanna's discussion of the notion of 'nature' in the work of Galen. Jouanna (2003b).

172 Gal. 2.343; trans. Singer (1996) 61; 8, 56;8, 213; *On Examining the Physician*, 9.9–13: *CMG* Suppl. Or. 4.106–109.

173 Nutton (2004) 236.

174 Ibid.

Like many other physicians, Galen emphasised the importance of securing the patient's trust. Following Hippocrates, he recommended accurate prognosis as the best possible way to achieve this trust.[175] Apparently such expertise was a rarity amongst Galen's contemporary physicians, unlike the situation among sacred healers. When he provided his prognosis he had difficulties persuading his audience that he was not a miracle worker, but a physician: ὥστε ἀγαπήσειεν ἄν, εἰ μὴ καὶ γόης τις εἶναι δόξειεν.[176] In order to obtain an accurate prognosis Galen first and foremost employed observation. Having once collected information he saw himself in a position to look for a cause.[177] Galen was aware of the ambiguity of causes and he was careful to distinguish between a primary external cause (e.g. an injury, bad nourishment, exposure to extreme temperatures etc.) and posterior causes (i.e. bodily procedures).[178] Having established a diagnosis and identified a causal chain, treatment could commence, with the intention of restoring the functional or humoral imbalance.[179]

Galen himself was conscious of the need for a clear understanding and explanation of the notions of health, disease and symptoms and the interrelations between them. In a 2006 study Ian Johnston has demonstrated how careful Galen was in addressing these three notions, both in themselves as well as the causal relations between them.[180] By looking into four of Galen's works Johnston classified Galen's terminology of health, disease and symptoms.[181] According to Galen, one cannot classify, or give an adequate account of the causes of disease and symptoms without initially defining and understanding what these terms mean.[182] In order to achieve this, a concept of health must also be apprehended and defined. Galen saw himself as a student of Plato here, at least from a methodological point of view. He argued that in order to take a comprehensive view, and bring under one form widely scattered particulars, the physician must have a

---

175 Gal. *Prog.* 14. 599 K = *CMG* 5.8.1 p. 69.

176 Gal. *Prog.* 14. 601 K = *CMG* 5.8.1; *On Examining the Physician* 4.4–5.19: *CMG* Suppl. Or. 4.64–79.

177 Barnes (1991).

178 The relevant evidence from Galen's work is collected and discussed in Hankinson (1998b) along with a broader discussion on causality in medicine amongst Greek scholars in Hankinson (1998a).

179 Gal. 18B.1–42 K.

180 Johnston (2006).

181 Gal. *The Differentiate of* Diseases; *The Causes of Diseases*; *The Differentiate of Symptoms*; *The Causes of Symptoms I–III*; Johnston (2006) 21–64.

182 Johnston (2006) 63.

definition of a healthy subject. Such a definition is instructive when examining a patient.[183]

Prior to these four Galenic treatises there had been no attempt to formulate an exhaustive nosology or a definition-system of all diseases and symptoms.[184] This absence is especially conspicuous in the Hippocratic Corpus, because its authors were noticeably influenced by the sophistic movement, which in itself paid much attention to definitions and classifications.[185] Plato's *Timaeus* attempts to classify diseases, although, as in the Hippocratic Corpus, it is without distinction between diseases and symptoms and without prior definitions.[186] Another attempt to formulate a classification of diseases appears at the outset of Celsus' third book on medicine. Celsus divided diseases into two categories, chronic and acute, claiming this division to be of Greek origin.[187] Celsus, though not without reservation towards this taxonomy, accepts its logic, which is a distinction between long term diseases and those of a short span. A similar taxonomy also appears in Caelius Aurelianus' compendium of diseases.[188] Thus, prior to Galen there were no systematic attempts to define disease or symptom (although Aristotle does give some thought to the definition of health)[189] nor to draw a distinction between health and disease or between disease, symptom and affection. Nor were there any systematic attempts to provide a complete classification of diseases and symptoms, either separately or jointly. All that could be claimed is that there were some attempts at rearrangement of material on diseases and symptoms considered jointly and organised, if at all, topographically.[190]

According to Galen the definition of health and disease rests on three terms: (i) condition/constitution (διάθεσις/ κατασκευή), (ii) function (ἐνέργεια), and (iii) whether or not something is in accordance with/against nature (κατὰ/ παρὰ φύσιν).[191] Health, therefore, is properly constituted parts of the body carrying out their appointed functions in accordance with nature. Disease is a diversion from this state of affairs. A proper condition

183 Gal. 9.5.15 K, quoting Pl. *Phdr.* 256d.
184 These four works of Galen considered three aspects of diseases and their symptoms: (i) definition (ii) classification (iii) causation. Johnston (2006) 65.
185 Lonie (1981) 328–329.
186 Johnston (2006) 66.
187 Celsus, *Med.* 3.1.
188 Johnston (2006) 67.
189 Arist. *Top.* 106b34–107a2; 110a19–21.
190 Johnston (2006) 67.
191 Johnston (2006) 306.

is that of 'balance', which Galen believed to be the balance of the four humours (hot, cold, dry and wet).[192]

Although Galen identified certain groups of symptoms, which he later associated with particular diseases, the treatments he prescribed were by no means general. In fact, Galen attacked the Methodists for prescribing the same treatment for all patients with similar symptoms.[193] Nutton has noted how Galen composed relatively little work on disease as such, and preferred to focus on the way in which each part of the body functioned and to examine symptoms and processes of illnesses.[194]

The actual therapeutic measures Galen prescribed included letting blood from a vein, herbal drugs, diet and certain physical activities. Surgery, on the other hand, was undesirable. The best physician is the one who knows how to achieve by diet and drugs what less able physicians achieve with a knife.[195] Diet was particularly important and Galen believed it should encompass not merely food and drink, but also lifestyle, sleep and exercise.

Inscriptions and works of other Greek authors, such as Plutarch and Lucian, help us to see Galen in a wider context. It appears that his choice of medicine as a vocation was not exceptional in the upper class of Asia Minor; neither was rising to the heights of either Greek civic or imperial ranks via a medical career.[196] Galen embodied the Greek world of his day in other ways as well. He was a keen advocate of Greek *paideia* and shared many characteristics with his contemporary Greek sophists. Although he lived in Rome for most of his life, his work and cultural world remained fundamentally Greek. Another noteworthy Greek physician who had achieved success in Rome almost a century before Galen was Caius Stertinius Xenophon, who acquired great wealth in the court of Claudius. Born into the Asclepiad family on the island of Cos, Xenophon gained Roman citizenship and travelled to Rome for the purpose of practising medicine. His wealth did not come exclusively from the imperial house, but also from his service in the fashionable spa resort, Baiae, on the north side of the bay of Naples. He was influential enough to promote the interests of Greeks and his native Cos in particular.[197] Through the pleas of Xenophon Claudius

---

192 Ibid.

193 Gal. 10.370 K.

194 Nutton (2004) 239, with reference to Gal. 7.766–804 K.

195 Gal. *On Examining the Physician* 10.1: *CMG* Suppl. Or. 4.116–117.

196 Nutton (2004) 256–257.

197 On Stertinius Xenophon see: Buraselis (2000) 66–110; Sherwin-White (1978) 149–152, 283–285.

exempted the island from paying tax and the temple of Asclepius reached the peak of its prosperity.[198]

By examining both the ancient explanations and vocabulary of disease it has become clear that classical antiquity entertained no rigid distinction between scientific medicine and religious explanations of illness. The near contemporary of Aristides Hyginus could mix medical vocabulary and mythology when explaining that *Chiron Centaurus Saturni filius autem medicinam chirurgicam ex herbis primus instituit; Apollo autem oracularіam (Craik, codd. Ocularіam) medicinam primus fecit; tertio autem loco Asclepius Apollonis filius clinicem repperit.*[199] In addition, two of the most common methods of healing, namely by cleansing and by drugs, exemplified the fact that the choice between comprehending disease on a physiological level or as atonement lay in the eyes of the beholder, it was not determined by the therapeutic act itself. Likewise, the use of medical vocabulary in a political context cannot exclude the possibility that it was not done metaphorically, but due to an understanding of the nature of disease that is substantially different to the one that we hold today. The various medical schools in the Graeco-Roman world and the identity of its leading physicians which have been discussed in this section will provide the points of reference for a contextualisation of the experiences Aristides recorded in the *Sacred Tales*. Furthermore, this review of the Greek influence on Roman medicine (both in terms of medical theories and practices and in terms of religious healing and the cult of Asclepius) reveals that Aristides' choices of who to approach for health-care (either physicians or gods) were neither alien to his contemporary Romans nor frowned upon by them. His thoughts and deeds, which seemed eccentric to modern scholars, appear more orthodox when contextualised.

Dreams

According to the *Sacred Tales*, dreams had a seminal role in Aristides' medical treatment. Asclepius habitually sent Aristides dreams which contained medical advice.[200] Aristides and those around him, physicians and priests

---

198 Tac. *Ann.* 12. 61, 67; Plin. *NH.* 29.5.7; Jackson (1988) 56; Nutton (2004) 254–255.

199 Chiron the Centaur, son of Saturn, initially set surgical medicine out of herbs; then Apollo first made oracular medicine; in the third place Asclepius, son of Apollo discovered clinical medicine; Hyg. *Fab.* 274.9.

200 As noted above, this view was also taken by Galen and was attested by him to be widely accepted, p. 63.

alike, acknowledged the divine nature of these dreams and therefore the medical rationale of following the regimen they prescribed. In this section I will look into the ways dreams were understood in classical antiquity; their medical and religious use; and how such a consideration provides the necessary basis for a reading of the *Sacred Tales* themselves.[201]

The elusive nature of ancient medicine and its connection with other therapeutic methods, notably the magical or religious, was nowhere more acute than in the Graeco-Roman approach towards dreams and the stimulation of dreams as part of a medical treatment,[202] frequently by incubation (χρηματισμός Artem. 1.2. Macr. *Scip.* 1.3.2. Other common expressions are: ἐγκαθεύδειν, ἐγκοιμίζειν, ἐγκατακοιμίσθαι, ἐπικαταγκοιμίσθαι, ἐγκοιμίζειν, ἐγκοιμᾶσθαι,). Incubation meant sleeping with the intention of receiving prophecy. It is a ritual sleeping in order to obtain a dream, mostly for healing. Incubation was extensively practised in the sanctuaries of Asclepius,[203] but also in other healing sanctuaries such as that of Amphiaraus at Oropus or the oracular shrines like the Daunian ones of Calchas,[204] and Podalirius.[205] Sarapis and Isis also cured through dreams and incubation was practised in their temples as well. Furthermore, in the temple of Sarapis in Delos there were ὀνειροκρίται, professional dream-interpreters.[206] Votive offerings in the form of eyes made out of silver and gold suggest that eye treatment was offered there.[207] In these temples patients spent the night in sleeping-halls specially designated for this purpose.[208] The Epidaurian *iamata*, stelai displayed in the sleeping hall (*abaton*) which included details from previous miraculous cures, provide an excellent testimony to the cures Asclepius pro-

[201] Though there have been some attempts to look at Aristides' dreams from the point of view of modern (i.e. post-Freudian) psychology I will not engage with these issues here. There are two reasons for this suspension of judgement: the first is that I am not a trained psychologist and the second is that the reservations raised by the unjustified claim for universality of modern psychology and its approach to dreams as well as the obvious absence of the 'patient' himself from the psychologist's couch pose insurmountable difficulties. For other views see: Michenaud and Dierkens (1972) and Hazard-Guillon (1983).

[202] Cf. Pelling (1997) 197; Cox Miller (1994) 106–123.

[203] Testimonies are collected in Edelstein and Edelstein vol. i (1945) T 414–442.

[204] Str. 6.3.9.

[205] Lyc. *Alex.* 1050. See also Petsalis-Diomidis (2006b) 205–229.

[206] *I. Delos* 2071, 2072, 2073, 2105, 2110, 2120, 2151, 2619.

[207] Cox Miller (1994) 110; Griffiths (1978) 139, 236–237. Eye votives should probably be interpreted literally, that is referring to eye problems rather than as a reference to seeing the god in a dream because they are only one example in a whole spectrum of votives depicting bodily parts in the healing sanctuaries. These bodily parts often allude to a medical problem. Cf. Van Straten (1981); Petsalis-Diomidis (2010) Fig. 78, 79, 80.

[208] Hoffmann (1998) 55 and fig. 3.

vided, as well as to the widespread appeal of the cult.[209] A vivid description of such a night of incubation is that of Aristophanes.[210] Other sources of information are inscriptions and, of course, Aristides' *Sacred Tales*,[211] all of which were written with hindsight, after a dream vision from the god was delivered and a cure was procured.[212] The ritual of incubation followed preliminary cathartic rites and offerings. In the Athenian Asclepieion it was a bath in the sea,[213] and in other sanctuaries of Asclepius it was offerings of bloodless cakes, and for Amphiaraus, Podalirius, and Calchas it was a ram. In Pergamum Mnemosyne ('memory' in order to remember the dreams) was also among the recipients of offerings.[214]

Patricia Cox Miller analysed four examples of dream-induced therapy—two of which addressed physical ailments and the other two addressed mental illnesses—in order to demonstrate the wide-ranging use of dreams in therapy in classical antiquity.[215] Her first case-study is taken from Galen, and it concerned the cult of Asclepius and his temple in Pergamum. Galen wrote:

> ἄλλος δέ τις ἀνὴρ πλούσιος οὐχ ἡμεδαπὸς οὗτός γε, ἀλλ' ἐκ μέσης Θρᾴκης ἧκεν, ὀνείρατος προτρέψαντος αὐτὸν εἰς τὸ Πέργαμον, εἶτα τοῦ θεοῦ προστάξαντος ὄναρ αὐτῷ πίνειν τε τοῦ διὰ τῶν ἐχιδνῶν φαρμάκου καθ' ἑκάστην ἡμέραν καὶ χρίειν ἔξωθεν τὸ σῶμα, μετέπεσεν τὸ πάθος οὐ μετὰ πολλὰς ἡμέρας εἰς λέπραν, ἐθεραπεύθη τε πάλιν οἷς ὁ θεὸς ἐκέλευεν φαρμάκοις καὶ τοῦτο τὸ νόσημα.[216]

> Another wealthy man, this one not a native but from the interior of Thrace, came, because a dream had driven him, to Pergamum. Then a dream appeared to him, the god [Asclepius] prescribing that he should drink every

---

209 These inscriptions were re-edited by Lidonnici (1995). See also Furley and Bremer vol. i. (2001) 209. Dillon (1994) 239–260 discusses the nature of these *iamata*.

210 Ar. *Pl.* 653–747.

211 Harris commented that 'the most impressive evidence of all [for the common view of dreams as having predictive faculties] from the Roman Empire may be the large number of surviving inscriptions (there are nearly 400 of them, according to Gil Renberg, who recently made a special study of them for his doctoral dissertation) which state that so-and-so made a dedication because of a dream'. Harris (2003) 20.

212 Graf (1992) 186–193. For inscriptions from Pergamum see: Wörrle (1969), no. 161. The healing inscriptions: Müller (1987) 193–223. For a text from Amphipolis see: Véligianni (1994) 391 ff.

213 Ar. *Pl.* 656–658.

214 The process of pre-incubation and the way in which the visual surroundings of the Pergamene Asclepieion guided worshippers during their stay concerning both the practice within the temple and their expectations from it is discussed by Petsalis-Diomidis (2010) chap. 4.

215 Cox Miller (1994)106–123.

216 Gal. *Subfiguratio empirica*, Cp. 10, p. 78 [ed. Deichgräber].

> day of the drug produced from the vipers and should anoint the body from the outside. The disease after a few days turned into leprosy; and this disease, in turn, was cured by the drugs which the god commanded.

It is implicit in Galen's comments that the reputation of the Pergamene Asclepieion spread far and wide. A second interesting point is that Asclepius' vocabulary was also used by physicians (and vice versa). In particular, the use of drugs (φάρμακα) was common to physicians and Asclepius alike. As has been noted before,[217] φάρμακον meant a cure as well as a poison, and Galen here uses this term to mean both.[218] The fact that Asclepius prescribed the wealthy Thracian a drug made sense in both a medical and also a religious context. The myth of Asclepius linked him with Chiron, the wise centaur, who was skilled in the knowledge of drugs and lived on Mount Pelion which was renowned for its herbs.[219] Being skilful in the use of drugs was, therefore, expected of Asclepius.

Another testimony from Galen describes how popular the cult of Asclepius was in Asia Minor and how common it was for Asclepius to prescribe his worshippers therapeutic measures through dreams. Furthermore, as we shall later see, some of these prescriptions must have been quite popular and were also prescribed to Aristides himself.[220] Galen writes:

> οὐκ ὀλίγας μὲν ᾠδάς τε γράφεσθαι καὶ μίμους γελοίων καὶ μέλη τινὰ ποιεῖν ἐπιτάξας, οἷς αἱ τοῦ θυμοειδοῦς κινήςεις σφοδρότεραι γενόμεναι θερμοτέραν τοῦ δέοντος ἀπειργάζοντο τὴν κρᾶσιν τοῦ σώματος, ἑτέροις δέ τισιν, | οὐκ ὀλίγοις οὐδὲ τούτοις, κυνηγετεῖν καὶ ἱππάζεσθαι καὶ ὁπλομαχεῖν. εὐθὺς δὲ τούτοις διώρισε τό τε τῶν κυνηγεσίων εἶδος, οἷς τοῦτο προσέταξε, τό τε τῆς ὁπλίσεως, οἷς δι' ὅπλων ἐκέλευσε τὰ γυμνάσια ποιεῖσθαι. οὐ γὰρ μόνον ἐπεγείρειν αὐτῶν τὸ θυμοειδὲς ἐβουλήθη, ἄρρωςτον ὑπάρχον, ἀλλὰ καὶ μέτρον ὡρίςατο τῇ τῶν γυμναςίων ἰδέᾳ.[221]

> And not a few men, however many years they were ill through the disposition of their souls, we have made healthy by correcting the disproportion of their emotions. No slight witness of that statement is our ancestral god Asclepius who ordered not a few to have odes written as well as to compose comical

[217] Pp. 44–49.

[218] Surely a drug made out of vipers was likely to have been poisonous. By using it the patient showed his confidence in Asclepius and in the physicians who medicated him and sanctioned the interpretation of his dream as a divine message.

[219] Cf. Pind. *Pyth*. 3.1–58; Ov. *Met*. 2.542–648; Apollod. *Bibl*. 3.10.3.5–4.1; Theodoretus, *Graecarum affectionum curatio*, 8.19–23.

[220] This means that either Asclepius himself prescribed the same regimen for more than one patient, or that more than one patient (maybe after learning that other patients received this prescription from Asclepius and were healed) expected to have received this particular regimen from the god.

[221] Gal. *De sanitate tuenda*, 1.8.19–21.

> mimes and certain songs (for the motion of their passions, having become more vehement, made the temperature of the body warmer than it should be); and for others, these not a few either, he ordered hunting and horse riding and exercising in arms; and at the same time he set a limit to the kind of hunting for those whom he prescribed this ... For he not only desired to awake the passion of these men because it was weak but also defined measure by the form of exercises.

It thus appears that a distinguished physician such as Galen regularly used dreams in his practice, and that he did not draw a dichotomy between mental problems and physiological ones. Furthermore, these views were long lasting, and Cox Miller refers to two later examples, one from Augustine's day and another from Abba Elias', which demonstrate that a Christianised form of therapy through dreams still existed in late antiquity.[222]

Incubation and the inducement of dreams for medical purposes are meaningful only if a certain understanding of the nature of dreams prevails. One has to acknowledge that the god 'reveals himself in person to man' (καὶ ὁ 'Ασκληπιὸς αὐτος ἐπιδήλος τοῖς ἀνθρώποις)[223] in a dream and that the dream itself is not a creation of the dreamer, but rather that it is delivered to him by the god.[224] In the Graeco-Roman world it was common in the dream experience to see the dream figure as existing objectively in space, and independent of the dreamer.[225] The Greeks never spoke of *having* a dream but of *seeing* a dream.[226] They also distinguished between significant dreams and non-significant ones.[227] In the category of the significant dreams several types were recognised. This classification, known to us through the works of Artemidorus, Macrobius and other authors, finds support in the works of authors as early as Homer who is familiar with at least three types of significant dreams. One is the symbolic dream, inaccessible without

---

222 August. De *civ. D.* 22.8.22; Palladius, *Lausiac History*, 29.4; Cox Miller (1994) 107–109.

223 Philostr. *VA* 1.7.

224 The large number of what Renberg has referred to as *viso/iussu* inscriptions proves that this was, indeed, a widespread belief. Nor was this view restricted to a certain province as becomes evident from the works of Müller (1987) regarding an inscription from Pergamum; Veyne (1987) in regards to Dalmatia; Palmer (1976) on an unusual dedication to Jupiter Fulgerator sought by the Dii Montenes in Rome; an *ex viso/iussu* dedication type to Jupiter from Rome was looked at by Cavallaro (1975–1976) and Palmer (1980) and Gamberale (1987) examined an *ex viso/iussu* from Africa; finally Marwood (1980) discussed a similar inscription from a British altar to the imperial cult. All these inscriptions have been collected in Renberg's (2003) catalogue.

225 Dodds (1951) 104.

226 Dodds (1951) 105.

227 For ancient systems of dream-classifications see Kessels (1969).

interpretation. The second type is the ὅραμα, or 'vision', which predicts a future event in a straightforward manner. The third type is called χρηματισμός or 'oracle', whereby in the sleep the dreamer's parent, or even a god, reveals without symbolism what will or will not happen, or should or should not be done.[228]

As a member of the educated upper class of the Greek world of Asia Minor, Aristides was likely to share this view about the nature of dreams and their function in medical practice. His particular affinity towards Asclepius, which was not unlikely to have been induced by his illness, would have further encouraged this view. This inclination of Aristides was not exceptional, particularly among the educated provinces of Greek society at this time. After all, Philostratus, the third century biographer of the sophists and hagiographer of Apollonius of Tyana, has the young philosopher-sage who embodied one extreme form of *pepaideumenos*-philosopher settle in Aegeae for his studies of philosophy next to the temple of Asclepius.[229] It appears that the temple was either a centre for philosophical studies itself or, at least, was closely connected to philosophical studies held nearby in Aegeae.[230]

The possibility of interaction directly with a deity in a variety of ways, and that such communication could be established via dreams, was a truism in Aristides' day.[231] Inscriptions and literary reports testify that the appearance of a deity in a dream bearing a command was common in the dream experience in the Graeco-Roman world.[232] Needless to say, at certain moments people are more receptive to messages in their dreams and even expect them. In the Asclepieia, for example, where the sick came to be healed by a deity that prescribed its treatment through dreams, all dreams were seen as god-sent, which made incubation highly efficient in the eyes of those present.[233] Of his own dreams Aristides says: 'For there was a seeming, as

228 Artem. 1.2. p. 4; Macrob. In *Somn.* 1.3.2; [Aug]. *de spiritu et anima*, 25 (*PL.* XL. 798); Joann. Saresb. *Polycart.* 2. 15 (*PL.* CXCIX. 429a); Nicephoros Gregoras, *in Synesium de insomn.* (*PG.* CXLIX. 608a). All these passages have been collected by Deubner, *De Incubatione.* The definitions quoted in the text are from Macrobius. See also the discussion in Dodds (1951) 124 n. 25.

229 Philostr. *VA* 1.7.

230 Hoffmann (1998) 51.

231 Gil Renberg collected 1300 inscriptions (623 in Greek and 677 in Latin) which cite a direct divine communication as the motivation for a dedication or some other undertaking. Renberg (2003) 1–7 and *passim*; see also Hanson (1980) 1395–1427.

232 *Syll*³ 663; 985; Pl. *Lg.* 909e–910a; Dodds (1951) 108. Van Straten (1976) collected no less than 225 votive-inscriptions, encouraged by an epiphany of a deity in a dream or a daydream.

233 Dodds (1951) 110–111.

it were, to touch him and to perceive that he himself had come, and to be between sleep and waking ... and to hear some things as in a dream, some as in a waking state'.[234] In the morning those whom the god visited during the night in their dreams shared the experience with the other worshippers/convalescents and with the temple-priests. Thus a supervised and regulated process of dream interpretation, which was an inherent aspect of life in the Asclepieia, helped patients to adopt a particular view of dreams and to conform to existing oneirocritical/medical traditions. Dodds explained this process using the Freudian notion of a 'secondary dream' which is the transformation of the dream-material into an intelligible, coherent, and communicable experience.[235] Aristides himself experienced no difficulties when discussing his dreams with others, and he had no problems convincing physicians that the god revealed himself to him in his dreams and prescribed him a trustworthy regimen.[236]

However, not all ancients shared this view of the meaning of dreams. More reserved opinions were also heard. Heraclitus maintained that in a dream each man enters into a world of his own.[237] The Hippocratic author of *On Regimen* 4 stressed that dreams can reflect the dreamer's current physiological and psychological state.[238] Aristotle in his treatises *On Dreams* and *On Divination in Sleep* denied any of the dreams to be god-sent.[239] Rather, Aristotle held that dreaming is a faculty of the soul, occurring during sleep with the dreamer its creator.[240] Moreover, since while asleep our judgement is not functioning, a perceptual fragment resembling a real one obtained by the sense-impressions is mistakenly thought to be real.[241] Such a view of the nature of dreams prohibited Aristotle from accepting what he acknowledged to be a commonly held view, namely that divination through dreams is possible.[242] But even Aristotle did not reject the importance of dreams in

---

234 αὐτὸς ἥκοι καὶ μέσως ἔχειν ὕπνου καὶ ἐγρηγόρσεως καὶ βούλεσθαι ἐκβλέπειν, καὶ ἀγωνιᾶν μὴ προαπαλλαγείη, καὶ ὦτα παραβεβληκέναι καὶ ἀκούειν, τὰ μὲν ὡς ὄναρ, τὰ δὲ ὡς ὕπαρ. Aristid. *Or.* 48. 32 K.

235 Dodds (1951) 114; Freud (1991) 391, defines a secondary dream by saying: 'that the dream loses the appearance of absurdity and incoherence, and approaches the pattern of an intelligible experience'.

236 Cf. Aristid. *Or.* 47. 57; 48. 34 K.

237 Heraclitus, *Fr.* 89 D; *Fr.* 73, and Sext. Emp. 1.129 (= Heraclitus, A 16). Dodds (1951) 131.

238 Hippoc. *Vict.* 86.

239 Arist. *Div. Somn.* 462b20–22, 463b12–14. Van Der Eijk (1995) discusses Aristotle's approach towards the medical use of dreams, a view he ascribed to certain 'distinguished physicians'.

240 Arist. *De Somn.* 459a14.

241 Arist. *De Somn.* 461b7–30.

242 Arist. *Div.Somn.* 462b12 is where he refers to such a common view.

the practice of medicine, and argued they were able to predict illness. 'Even medical experts' Aristotle claimed 'say that one should pay extremely close attention to dreams'.[243] This, however, is not due to a divine voice the dream allegedly carries, but because when asleep one is particularly attentive even to the smallest things and with them to any changes in his constitution.[244] This medical quality which Aristotle saw in dreams agrees with his previous argument that dreams are not sent by god.[245] 'For, apart from its general irrationality, the idea that it is god who sends [dreams], and yet that he sends them not to the best and most intelligent, but to random people, is absurd'.[246] In his concluding note in *On Divination through Sleep*, Aristotle defines the proper method of dream interpretation: 'the most skilled interpreter of dreams is one who can observe resemblances. For anyone can interpret a direct dream'.[247] Dreams, as Aristotle perceived them, were a creation of the dreamer's mind. They are meaningful and medically useful even if their origin is not divine.

All these various approaches to the understanding of the dream-mechanism made dreams highly relevant to the practice of medicine. The Hippocratic author of the treatise *On Regimen* 4 considered dreams as an inherent part of his subject matter. In the fourth part of his work he specifically discusses dreams: 'He who has learnt aright about the signs that come up in sleep will find that they have an important influence upon all things'.[248] As for their nature, this author held that certain dreams are godly and foretell the future of cities and individuals.[249] The meaning of these dreams was only accessible with the help of those who possessed the art of the interpretation of dreams. However, the dreamer was advised to consult a physician, not a dream interpreter, when the dreams concerned his physical symptoms.[250] The Hippocratic author of *On Regimen* 4, it appears, accepted both the view that certain dreams could be predictive, as well as the fact that

[243] λέγουσι γοῦν καὶ τῶν ἰατρῶν οἱ χαρίεντες ὅτι δεῖ σφόδρα προσέχειν τοῖς ἐυπνίοις. Arist. *Div.Somn.* 463a5.

[244] Arist. *Div.Somn.* 463b10–20.

[245] Arist. *Div.Somn.* 463b12–22.

[246] τό τε γὰρ θεὸν εἶναι τὸν πέμποντα, πρὸς τῇ ἄλλῃ ἀλογίᾳ, καὶ τὸ μὴ τοῖς βελτίστοις καὶ φρονιμωτάτοις ἀλλὰ τοῖς τυχοῦσι πέμπειν ἄτοπον. Arist. *Div.Somn.* 462b20.

[247] τεχνικώτατος δ' ἐστὶ κριτὴς ἐνυπνίων ὅστις δύναται τὰς ὁμοιότητας θεωρεῖν· τὰς γὰρ εὐθυονειρίας κρίνειν παντός ἐστιν. Arist. *Div.Somn.* 464b5–6.

[248] Περὶ δὲ τῶν τεκμηρίων τῶν ἐν τοῖσιν ὕπνοισιν ὅστις ὀρθῶς ἔγνωκε, μεγάλην ἔχοντα δύναμιν εὑρήσει πρὸς ἅπαντα. Hippoc. *Vict.* 86.

[249] Hippoc. *Vict.* 87.

[250] Ibid.

some dreams are natural faculties of the human body. The interpretation of each type fell under the jurisdiction of the diviner and the physician accordingly.

The content of dreams allows the Hippocratic physician to prescribe a regimen: 'now if the contrast [between the daily occurrences and the contents of the dream] be violent, it is beneficial to take an emetic, to increase gradually a light diet for five days, to take in the early morning long, sharp walks, increasing them gradually, and to adapt exercises, when in training, so as to match the gradual increase of food'.[251] Not all dreams are medically ominous. Some, in fact, signify good health. The Hippocratic author writes: 'They signify health because the soul abides by the purposes of the day and is overpowered neither by surfeit nor by depletion nor by any attack from without. But when dreams are contrary to the acts of the day, and there occurs about them some struggle or triumph, a disturbance in the body is indicated'.[252] For the Hippocratic physician, it therefore appears, dreams which concern medical issues are but one of many bodily functions.

These Hippocratic views (and, indeed, Hippocratic medicine) were still pertinent in Aristides' day. Rufus of Ephesus, for example, a physician of the Flavian age, is another example of a physician who used dreams to form a diagnosis.[253] Rufus thought that dreams are symptomatic of malfunctioning humours. Rufus was altogether convinced that dream-images signify either good things or bad things, which occur to the dreamer, according to his/her humours in the body.[254] Even the great Galen thought that although some people ignored dreams and dismissed them as meaningless there is much a physician can learn from them. While Galen acknowledged that some people despised dreams, omens and portents, he, on the other hand, often made use of dreams for a diagnosis.[255]

Ancient dream-interpretation and its medical implications did not exist in a void. As we learn from the vocabulary and examples of the author of *On*

---

[251] Ἢν μὲν οὖν ἰσχυρὸν ᾖ τὸ ἐναντιωθὲν, ἔμετόν τε ξυμφέρει ποιήσασθαι, καὶ τοῖσι σιτίοισι κούφοισι προσάγειν ἐς ἡμέρας πέντε καὶ τοῖσι περιπάτοισιν ὀρθρίοισι πολλοῖσι καὶ ὀξέσιν ἐκ προσαγωγῆς χρέεσθαι, καὶ τοῖσι γυμνασίοισιν ἐπιγυμνάζεσθαι συμμέτροισι πρὸς τὴν προσαγωγὴν τῶν σιτίων. Hippoc. *Vict.* 88.

[252] ὑγείην γὰρ σημαίνει, διότι ἡ ψυχὴ παραμένει ἐν τοῖσιν ἡμερινοῖσι βουλεύμασιν, οὔτε πλησμονῇ τινι κρατηθεῖσα οὔτε κενώσει οὔτε ἄλλῳ οὐδενὶ ἔξωθεν προσπεσόντι. Ὅταν δὲ πρὸς τὰς ἡμερινὰς πρήξιας ὑπεναντίωται τὰ ἐνύπνια καὶ ἐγγίνηται περὶ αὐτέων ἡ μάχη ἢ νίκη, τοῦτο σημαίνει ταραχὴν ἐν τῷ σώματι. Hippoc. *Vict.* 88.

[253] On this author see Abu Ali (1992).

[254] Rufus, *Medical Questions*, 5 (pp. 7–8 in the Teubner edn. by H. Gärtner).

[255] Gal. 16. 222 K.

Regimen 4, cosmology and astronomy, for instance, had much to contribute to medical oneirology 'to see the sun, moon, heavens and stars clear and bright, each in its proper order is good ... but if there be a contrast between the dream and reality, it indicates a physical illness, a violent contrast a violent illness, a slighter contrast a lighter illness'.[256] The Hippocratic author goes into some detail here on how it is possible to diagnose various illnesses in accordance with the particular disfigurement of the dream vision of the solar system. His perception of this system and of its meaning carried much weight in determining his medical diagnosis. The gods are no less relevant: 'So with this knowledge about the heavenly bodies, precaution must be taken, with change of regimen and prayers to the gods; in the case of good signs, to the Sun to Heavenly Zeus, to Zeus, Protector of Home, to Athena, Protectress of Home, to Hermes and Apollo; in the case of adverse signs, to the Averters of evil, to Earth and to the Heroes, that all dangers may be averted'.[257] This example demonstrates just how religiously-oriented the medical interpretation of dreams was, and how, according to this Hippocratic author, any dichotomy between medicine and religion was artificial.[258]

The Hellenistic physician, Herophilus of Alexandria, was also interested in the nature of dreams and, like his Hippocratic predecessors, he used dreams in his medical practice. Herophilus introduced a tripartite division of dreams, which, according to Heinrich Von Staden, 'seems to have launched a remarkably rich Hellenistic tradition of dream theory'.[259] Direct references to Herophilus' theory of dreams are found only in Aëtius and the pseudo-Galenic *De historia philosopha*. The latter, however, rests heavily on Aëtius or on a common source. Ps. Plutarch *Placita philosophorum* is identical to Aëtius. Von Staden finds traces of Herophilus' theory of dreams in

---

[256] Ἥλιον δὲ καὶ σελήνην καὶ οὐρανὸν καὶ ἀστέρας καθαρὰ καὶ εὐαγέα, κατὰ τρόπον ὁρεόμενα ἕκαστα, ἀγαθά· ὑγείην γὰρ τῷ σώματι σημαίνει ἀπὸ πάντων τῶν ὑπαρχόντων· ἀλλὰ χρὴ διαφυλάσσειν ταύτην τὴν ἕξιν τῇ παρούσῃ διαίτῃ. Εἰ δέ τι τούτων ὑπεναντίον γένοιτο, νοῦσόν τινα τῷ σώματι σημαίνει, ἀπὸ μὲν τῶν ἰσχυροτέρων ἰσχυροτέρην, ἀπὸ δὲ τῶν ἀσθενεστέρων κουφοτέρην. Hippoc. *Vict.* 89. For the cosmological applications of the dream theory in the treatise *On Regimen* see Jouanna (1998).

[257] Περὶ μὲν οὖν τῶν οὐρανίων σημείων οὕτω χρὴ γινώσκοντα προμηθέεσθαι καὶ ἐκδιαιτῆσθαι καὶ τοῖσι θεοῖσιν εὔχεσθαι, ἐπὶ μὲν τοῖσιν ἀγαθοῖσιν Ἡλίῳ, Διὶ οὐρανίῳ, Διὶ κτησίῳ, Ἀθηνᾷ κτησίῃ, Ἑρμῇ, Ἀπόλλωνι, ἐπὶ δὲ τοῖσιν ἐναντίοισι τοῖσιν ἀποτροπαίοισι, καὶ Γῇ καὶ ἥρωσιν, ἀποτρόπαια γενέσθαι τὰ χαλεπὰ πάντα. Hippoc. *Vict.* 89.

[258] The author of *Hippoc. Vict.* was probably the author of *The Sacred Disease* as well: Jouanna (1999) 374–375.

[259] Von Staden (1989) 307–308.

Poseidonius,[260] the Stoics,[261] and Philo.[262] Patristic authors, such as Tertullian,[263] Prudentius,[264] Cassianus,[265] and St. Augustine[266] were also influenced by Herophilus' approach towards the nature of dreams. Herophilus' theory of dreams included a category of god-sent dreams and another category of dreams which result from bodily activity.[267] It is only the latter category which interested him as a physician. Aëtius has the following text (= Ps. Plut. *Placita Philosophorum* 5.1.2 = Von Staden T 226a–b):

> Ἡρόφιλος τῶν ὀνείρων τοὺς μὲν θεοπνεύστους κατ' ἀνάγκην γίνεσθαι, τοὺς δὲ φυσικοὺς ἀνειδωλοποιουμένης τῆς ψυχῆς τὸ συμφέρον αὐτῇ καὶ τὸ πρὸς τούτοις ἐσόμενον, τοὺς δὲ συγκραματικοὺς ἐκ τοῦ αὐτομάτου κατ' εἰδώλων πρόσπτωσιν, ὅταν ἃ βουλόμεθα βλέπωμεν, ὡς ἐπὶ τῶν τὰς ἐρωμένας ἐχόντων ἐν ὕπνῳ γίνεται
>
> Herophilus says that some dreams are inspired by god, while others are natural ones and arise when the soul forms an image (*eidōlon*) of what is to its own advantage and of what will happen next; and still others are mixed and arise spontaneously [or 'accidentally'] according to the impact of the images, whenever we see what we wish, as happens in the case of those who in their sleep make love to the women they love.

The pseudo-Galenic treatise, *De historia Philosopha* 106 (= Von Staden T226c) is identical to the testimony of Aëtius:

> Ἡρόφιλος τῶν ὀνείρων τοὺς μὲν θεοπέμπτους κατ' ἀνάγκην γίγνεσθαι, τοὺς δὲ φυσικοὺς εἰδωλοποιουμένης τῆς ψυχῆς τὸ συμφέρον αὐτῇ καὶ τὸ πάντως ἐσόμενον· τοὺς δὲ συγκριματικοὺς αὐτομάτως κατ' εἰδώλων πρόσπτωσιν, ὅταν ἃ βουλόμεθα βλέπωμεν, <ὡς ἐπὶ τῶν> φιλούντων γίγνεται τὰς ἐρωμένας ἐρώντων ἐν ὕπνοις.
>
> Herophilus says that some dreams are sent by god and arise by necessity, while others are natural and arise when the soul makes for itself an image (*eidōlon*) of what is to its advantage and of what will undoubtedly happen; but the 'compound' dreams [arise] spontaneously, according to the impact of the images whenever we see what we wish, as happens in the case of men who harbour affection, when in their dreams they make love to the women they love.

It is clear from both passages that Herophilus followed the Hippocratic tradition of *Vict.* 87 and divided dreams into mantic and non-mantic.

---

260 Fr. 108 Edelstein/Kidd = Cic. *De Div.* 1.64.
261 Cf. SVF III. 605; SVF II. 1198.
262 Philo, *De insomniis*, 1.1–2; 2.1–4.
263 Tert. *De anima*, 47.
264 Prudentius, *Cathemerinon liber*, 6.37–40, 73–76, 137–140.
265 Johannes Cassianus, *Collectiones Patrum*, 1.19.
266 St. Aug. *Ep.* 162.5.9.3; *Civ. Dei.* 18.18.2; *De Trinitate*, 11.7.
267 Von Staden (1989) 306–310.

Hippocrates reserved the interpretation of mantic dreams to the dream interpreter but maintained that the other category, namely dreams which result from bodily activities, are pertinent for medical diagnosis and belong under the physician's jurisdiction rather than that of the dream-interpreter.[268] Kessels argued convincingly for a clear influence of Herophilus on Galen's view of dreams referring to the following text:

> ἐπεὶ δὲ ἐν τοῖς ὕπνοις οὐκ ἐπὶ ταῖς τοῦ σώματος ἡ ψυχὴ διαθέσεσι φαντάζεται μόνον, ἀλλὰ κᾀκ τῶν συνήθως ἡμῖν πραττομένων ὁσημέραι, ἔνια δὲ ἐξ ὧν πεφροντίκαμεν, καὶ δή τινα μαντικῶς ὑπ' αὐτῆς προδηλοῦνται, (καὶ γὰρ τοῦτο τῇ πείρᾳ μαρτυρεῖται,) δύσκολος ἡ διάγνωσις τοῦ σώματος γίγνεται ἐκ τῶν ἀπὸ τοῦ σώματος ὁρμωμένων ἐνυπνίων.[269]
>
> because the soul places [images] in dreams before one's mind not only in accordance to the dispositions of the body, but also out of our daily occurrences, and still other [images] out of our anxieties, while others are plainly seen by the soul as something of divination (which is testified by experience) it is troublesome to produce a diagnosis of the body out of dreams which are created by the body.

From this passage it is clear that Galen thought certain dreams are valuable for diagnosis and that he acknowledged the existence of mantic dreams. By dividing dreams into mantic and non-mantic Galen follows Herophilus and the Hippocratic author of *Vict.* Galen saw the role of the professional dream-interpreter to complete his role as a physician.

Any study of the importance of dreams in the Graeco-Roman world of the second century CE, and their relevance to medicine, cannot be fully undertaken without referring to Artemidorus. Born in Ephesus,[270] he wrote many other works, which are now lost, before composing his work on dreams in the mid- to late-second century.[271] Artemidorus divided his work into five books, of which the first three he dedicated to one Cassius Maximus.[272] The first two books are organised systematically by subject-matter. The third book is a supplement, explaining points which Artemidorus assumed a professional already knows.[273] The fourth book, which Artemidorus addressed

---

268 Hippoc. *Vict.* 87.

269 Gal. 6.833 K; Kessels (1969) 422–424.

270 Although Artemidorus himself was born in Ephesus he called himself 'of Daldis', which was his mother's native city in Lydia. It was Daldis' chief god, Apollo, who encouraged Artemidorus to compose his work on dreams.

271 Price (2004) 233.

272 It is, most-likely, the same Maximus of Tyre whose rhetorical works we still have today. Price (2004) 233.

273 Artem. 3.66, p. 234 1.4.

to his son as a guide-book for prospective professional dream-interpreter, is another supplement. The fifth book consists of ninety-five dreams which were known to have come true.[274] Artemidorus' main interest in dreams lay in their ability to predict the future. Not all dreams could have this capacity, and Artemidorus drew a distinction between dreams with predictive force (ὄνειροι), and those indicative only as to the present state of affairs (ἐνύπνια).[275] Predictive dreams, which included visions and oracular dreams, so Artemidorus explains, divide into two subcategories: dreams that predict the future directly (θεωρηματικοί) and those which predict the future allegorically (αλληγορικοί).[276] Although Artemidorus' primary interest was not medicine, he has numerous examples of dreams which predict medical problems, portray the medical advice of a god, or are a sign of a medical problem. Behr undertook a comparative study of the dream-symbols which are included in Artemidorus' work and Aristides' *Sacred Tales*. His results demonstrate a considerable agreement on specifics and on generalities between the two authors, such as the evaluation of the role of certain dream-figures.[277]

The existence of predictive dreams was widely accepted in antiquity. Aristides himself records a god-sent dream predicting the time of his death.[278] Moreover the terminology used by Artemidorus was not his own invention.[279] Indeed, χρηματισμοί had already been the subject of treatises composed by Artemon of Miletus,[280] Demetrius of Phalerum and Geminus of Tyre, and although χρηματισμός may not have been found in the early papyri χρηματίζω is clearly used to describe dreams which predicted the future.[281] Price has noted that 'there were numerous other Greek classifications of dreams by poets, philosophers, and medical writers, but almost all of these in various ways allowed for the existence of special predictive dreams'.[282] Artemidorus' main concern was to produce useful tools for the

274 Price (2004) 233.

275 Artem. 1.1. p. 3 (Citations of Artemidorus are by book and chapter numbers, adding the page number from the edition by R. Pack [Leipzig, 1963]).

276 Artem. 1.2. p, 4.

277 Behr (1968) 196–204.

278 Aristid. *Or.* 48. 18 K.

279 Deubner (1900) 1–4; Kessels (1969) 393–396.

280 Artem. 323, 21 Pack.

281 Cf. *IG* XII 2.108; *Pap. Cair. Zen.* 59034 (dated 257 B.C) lines 4–5 with Fraser (1960) 1–54; *IG* XI 4.1299 (about 200 B.C) line 13; *Pap. Par.* 3209; Kessels (1969) 394, mentions other instances of the use of the verb [4]: Aristid. 50.5 K; Jos. *Ant.* 11.327.

282 Price (2004) 235.

interpretation of dreams. He argued that, 'the interpretation of dreams is nothing other than the juxtaposition of similarities' (καὶ γὰρ οὐδὲν ἄλλο ἐστὶν ὀνειροκρισία ἢ ὁμοίου παράθεσις).[283] Naturally his work also contained some more practical guidelines. For example, he stated that only fully remembered dreams can be interpreted,[284] and that the interpreter has to know everything about the dreamer.[285] Artemidorus also thought that predictive dreams came from the gods, and was convinced that the gods could be encouraged to send such dreams.[286]

Artemidorus' treatise contains a long section on the interpretation of the appearances of particular gods in a dream.[287] In a religious society it is only natural that the gods form an important part of the dream-material. Moreover, Graeco-Roman visual culture introduced a canonised image of the various gods through works of visual art, which meant that a notion of a certain deity in classical antiquity was often intrinsically associated with a particular visual image of that god.[288] Like other predictive dreams those in which the gods appear also divide into direct and allegorical dreams. It is noteworthy, Artemidorus explains, that divine remedies are always direct.[289] The gods are trustworthy: 'the gods, I say, are first among those things which are said to be worthy of credence and whose words one must believe and obey; for lying is contrary to the nature of a god' (Τῶν δὲ ἀξιοπίστων λεγομένων, οἷς λέγουσι τι [κατ' ὄναρ] πιστεύειν χρὴ καὶ πείθεσθαι, φημὶ πρώτους εἶναι θεούς· ἀλλότριον γὰρ θεοῦ τὸ ψεύδεσθαι).[290] Such advice, coming from a professional dream-interpreter and contemporary of Aristides, is therefore highly valuable when trying to evaluate and contextualise Aristides' reactions to the dreams Asclepius sent him as they are recorded in the *Sacred Tales*.

A contextual approach to Artemidorus, so argues Price, can reveal hidden connections between interpretations of dreams and medicine. Artemidorus borrowed patterns of thinking from contemporary medical thought. As noted above, at this time there were three schools of medicine: Empiricists, Rationalists, and Methodists. They offered different and incompatible approaches to medicine as we learn from the conversation in Galen's dia-

---

[283] Artem. 2.25, p. 145.
[284] Artem. 1.12, p. 20; 1.18, p. 26; 4.3. p. 247.
[285] Artem. 1.9, pp. 18–19.
[286] Artem. 4.2, p. 246 1; 4.22, p. 255; Price (2004) 239.
[287] Artem. 2.33–39, pp. 155–176.
[288] See chapter 3, section 4, 'visual culture and social forms of cult-organisation' below.
[289] Artem. 4.22. p, 255 1.9; Price (2004) 242.
[290] Artem. 2.69. p, 195.

logue, *On Medical Experience*.[291] The Empiricists stressed the importance of experiment; reason was key for the Rationalists; and the Methodists argued that medicine was 'knowledge of manifest commonalities'. Artemidorus himself was clearly influenced by the Empiricist school and the three main elements of the Empiricist approach to medical knowledge—tradition (ἱστορία), analogy (μετάβασις τοῦ ὁμοῦ), and primarily experience (πεῖρα or τήρησις),[292] which constituted Artemidorus' own approach to the interpretation of dreams.

To conclude, in classical antiquity dreams were habitually seen as existing objectively rather than being viewed as a creation of the dreamer's mind. It was, therefore, meaningful to speak of dreams as a means of communication between gods and humans. Physicians were particularly interested in deciphering the dream-mechanism, both because of their general interest in the structure of human cognition and bodily faculties, and because of the utility of the information they hold for medical purposes. Using Kleinman's vocabulary, dreams were part of the Graeco-Roman health care system because their content was thought to be indicative of the dreamer's constitution. In turn, those who were approached to interpret them must have been those marked by that health care system as most able to do so. This authority, Barton explains, is revealing both as to the nature of therapeutic authority in classical antiquity and as to the power structure in the field of health care. All ancient commentators acknowledged the medical use of dreams in therapy, even those who did not accept their role in divination. They have thus hinted as to the grid of knowledge on which the health care system was founded, and in which Aristides operated. Dreams were also significant in the context of religion, mainly healing cults and predicting the future. However, in their use of dreams classical practitioners of medicine were often at no variance with dream-interpreters such as Artemidorus, his predecessors and successors. Furthermore, it would be misleading to depict a dichotomy between ancient approaches to the dream-phenomenon and its practical implications expressed by physicians and that of the diviner. Most Graeco-Roman physicians perceived the human body as a part of a larger system of nature and the cosmos. However, unlike modern scientific views, Graeco-Roman medicine did not include an empiricist component of trial and error, nor did it set a clear boundary between medical and physical questions and questions of cosmology, religion and myth. In this respect,

291 Price (2004) 246.
292 Price (2004) 246–253.

dreams containing medical information about cures and regimens were but one example of a divine message and their language and validity were identical to any other.

2. The Sick, Medicine and Physicians in the World of the *Sacred Tales*

A study of the sick, medicine and physicians, which is based on the *Sacred Tales*, has many obstacles to overcome. Aristides himself did not write the *Tales* as a medical treatise or as a general and critical survey of medicine at his time. On the contrary, he proclaimed that he had written the *Sacred Tales* as a eulogy to a benevolent god who saved him from the grip of disease.[293] All comments relevant to a study of medicine and the sick in society were made by Aristides either in passing or as parts of arguments of a different sort. Whilst acknowledging these limitations, the *Sacred Tales* do record many episodes in which Aristides encounters health-care providers (both men and gods). The *Sacred Tales* also provide an opportunity to learn how illness was conceived of; whom the world of the *Sacred Tales* denoted as authoritative in offering medical care; and the traits health-care providers were expected to have. In other words, the *Sacred Tales* can be read as what Geertz defined as a map of a cultural system within the field of health care. The *Sacred Tales* also name some of Aristides' physicians and other health-care providers, hence providing valuable personal information about those practising medicine.

This section of the chapter will therefore discuss the depiction of the sick, medicine and physicians in the *Sacred Tales*. In the first part I will examine the place of the sick in the world of the *Sacred Tales* and the attitude of society towards them. More specifically, I will be interested to learn whether the sick were seen as an inherent part of society or whether they were confined to its margins. Secondly, in the main part of the section I will try and determine if the world of the *Sacred Tales* had a discernable medical discourse by borrowing Wittgenstein's critical tools and looking into the meaning and the use of some key themes such as the identity of the health-care providers, the language they used and the procedures they prescribed. The final part of the section will examine the identity of the physicians themselves, with particular attention to their social standing.

293 Aristid. *Or.* 48.2–3 K.

The Place of the Sick in Society

The Pergamene Asclepieion, according to the *Sacred Tales*, was more of a social, religious and intellectual centre than a hospital.[294] With an impressive theatre, a library, and acting as a centre of worship it attracted a wide spectrum of visitors. Scholars like the philosopher Euarestus of Crete, whose acquaintance Aristides had already made while travelling in Egypt, arrived in the Pergamene Asclepieion not as patients, but in pursuit of knowledge of the god.[295] Not only scholars visited the temple, though. In August 146 CE Aristides was fortunate enough to meet the governor Julianus and the civic magnate Rufinus, who were both visiting the Asclepieion while healthy and well, and they offered Aristides some practical help with pending legal issues that troubled him.[296] Aristides also enjoyed the company of some distinguished scholars who were convalescing in the temple with him. They provided Aristides with valuable support in his decision to follow Asclepius' exhortation and resume the practice of oratory. Men like Salvius, of whom Aristides says that he is now a consul (Σαλβίου τοῦ νῦν ὑπάτου)[297] and Sedatius 'one of the Roman senators' (τινι τῶν ἐκ τῆς Ῥωμαίων βουλῆς),[298] provided Aristides with the moral encouragement and the intellectual stimulus he needed in order to resume declaiming. The *Sacred Tales*' account of Aristides' first attempt to resume oratory, in the autumn of 145 CE, has Aristides and Sedatius sitting in the temple of Hygieia in the Asclepieion complex and analysing Asclepius' command that Aristides should declaim again. It is not a picture of two men living on the margins of society. Rather, it is a description of an open, vibrant and intellectual environment, an impression which is further augmented by the fact that another distinguished scholar, one Maximus the African, joins the two, offering Aristides a theme for his oration.[299] Moreover, while this discussion takes place the vast majority of convalescents were not in the temple but in the city of Pergamum itself, enjoying a spectacle.[300]

---

294 I use the term 'hospital' loosely here, referring to a congregation of the sick and health-care providers in an institution which aimed to offer health-care.

295 Aristid. *Or.* 50.23 K.

296 Aristid. *Or.* 50.106–107 K.

297 Aristid. *Or.* 48.9 K. For the identity of Salvius see chapter 1 'date of composition' above, 14–15.

298 Aristid. *Or.* 48.48, 50.16 K.L. Sedatius Theophilus was a citizen of Nicaea on the Cayster and Laodiceia ad Lycum and was of praetorian rank. Bowersock (1969) 86–87; Behr (1981–1986) ad loc.

299 Aristid. *Or.* 50.16–18 K.

300 Aristid. *Or.* 50.16 K.

Medical Discourse in the Sacred Tales

Medical Authority

The *Sacred Tales* clearly identify a discernable set of health-care providers. They are recognised by their vocation, title and position.[301] Whenever Aristides needed medical care his first appeal was always to physicians. Be it in Rome, Smyrna, Macedonia or Thrace, Aristides never lost faith in the ability of physicians to help him,[302] even if their efforts were often found lacking. Later, when Aristides was ill during the summer of 165 CE, probably a result of the great plague, he was treated by physicians from Smyrna. Therefore although the narrative of the *Sacred Tales* was mainly concerned with the power of the god through telling of Aristides' miraculous recuperation, it appears that Aristides' appeals for medical help constantly extended to physicians. At no point in the *Sacred Tales* is there an episode of illness where physicians are altogether absent. Moreover, it is implicit in the narrative that the title 'physician' (ἰατρός) would be a familiar and specific enough term for its readers because no other attribute is added when denoting it.

Aristides did not turn to physicians because he was personally acquainted with them. On the contrary, he made their acquaintance because he sought the expertise their vocation and title suggested they possessed. His willingness to entrust himself to their hands and knives serves as powerful evidence in support of the reliable reputation of the title 'physician' (ἰατρός).[303] Furthermore, when Aristides learned that the daughter of his foster-sister was dangerously ill during the winter of 166 CE, probably infected by the great plague, he sent her a physician.[304] His decision to entrust his foster-niece to the hands of unnamed physician also demonstrates that medicine, the medical establishment and physicians as its agents were trustworthy figures in his eyes.[305] The physician's anonymity

---

301 Physicians: Asclepiacus: Aristid. *Or.* 48.35 K; Heracleon: 48.20 K; Porphyrio: Aristid. *Or.* 47.57; 51.12, 24 K; Satyrus: Aristid. *Or.* 48.8–10 K; Theodotus: Aristid. *Or.* 47.13, 55, 56; 48.34; 50.21.38.42; 51.57 K; Unnamed physicians: Aristid. *Or.* 47.62–63, 67; 48.5, 20, 38, 39, 69; 51.9, 49–52 K; Egyptian physicians: Aristid. *Or.* 48.15 K; Mysian physicians: Aristid. *Or.* 47.73; 49.18–19 K; Roman physicians: Aristid. *Or.* 48.63 K.

302 Appeals to physicians: Rome: Aristid. *Or.* 48.63 K; Macedonia and Thrace: Aristid. *Or.* 48.5 K.

303 Cf. in Rome; Aristid. *Or.* 48.63 K.

304 ἀγγέλλεται ἡ τῆς τρόφου θυγάτηρ ἀσθενούσα καὶ ἔχουσα σφαλερῶς. κἀκείνῃ μὲν ἰατρὸν ἔπαμπον. 'It was reported to me that the daughter of my foster sibling was ill and in a dangerous condition. I sent a physician for her'. Aristid. *Or.* 51.19 K.

305 Aristides did not name these physicians or indicated in any way that he was familiar with them. It is likely that he did not know them because Aristides was in the habit of naming

indicates that for Aristides and his contemporaries the mere title ἰατρός was sufficient to vouch for one's capacity to offer medical care. Aristides himself trusted medicine as a discipline and in consequence, its individual agents, not the other way around.

Physicians, however, were not the only group designated by the *Sacred Tales* as suitable to offer health-care. At least two other groups are recognised as appropriate people for the sick to address. The first of these groups is gymnastic trainers and the second is the temple-staff of the Asclepieia, notably the temple wardens of the Pergamene Asclepieion.[306] It appears from the *Tales* that each member of these three groups obtained his authority to offer health-care from being a physician, a gymnastic trainer or a member of the temple staff, rather than endorsing his group with authority that originated from his own personal charisma.[307] Hence, the world of the *Sacred Tales* definitely had a health-care establishment,[308] with agents who mastered a discipline, practised a vocation and were considered reliable merely because they carried certain titles of affiliation.

The *Sacred Tales* convey little evidence about the relations between members of each of these three categories of health-care providers or within the groups themselves. The paucity of evidence and ephemeral discussions of issues of health-care and its establishment *per se* is due to the genre of the work and its author's intentions.[309] Some valuable pieces of evidence can, however, be found. Firstly, physicians, gymnastic trainers and the temple staff did not consider their knowledge in offering health-care to be mutually exclusive. When Aristides returned to Smyrna from Rome in 144 CE he consulted physicians and gymnastic trainers together. The long narrative of

---

his physicians; cf. pp. 103–105 above. On the theme of physicians failing Aristides see Petsalis-Diomidis (2010).

306 Gymnastic trainers: Aristid. *Or.* 48.69 K; Temple wardens: Asclepiacus: Aristid. *Or.* 47. 58, 76, 48. 35 K; Philadelphus: Aristid. *Or.* 48.30, 31, 35, 47; 50.46 K.

307 The term charisma was introduced in scholarly usage by the German sociologist Max Weber. Weber defined charismatic authority to be one of three forms of authority, the other two being traditional (feudal) authority and legal or rational authority. According to Weber, charisma is defined thus: A certain quality of an individual personality, by virtue of which s/he is 'set apart' from ordinary people and treated as endowed with supernatural, superhuman, or at least specifically exceptional powers or qualities. These as such are not accessible to the ordinary person, but are regarded as divine in origin or as exemplary, and on the basis of them the individual concerned is treated as a leader.

308 'Establishment' in the sense that health-care activity was regulated and managed by social institutions, which were the relevant centres of power.

309 See the chapter 'Aelius Aristides and the *Sacred Tales*' for a discussion of the composition of the *Sacred Tales*.

his recuperation under Asclepius' supervision is interwoven with episodes of consultations with physicians, often working with one of the temple staff, while Aristides was still convalescing in a temple.[310] When a tumour grew 'from no apparent cause' (ἀπ' ἀρχῆς οὐδεμιᾶς φανερᾶς)[311] on Aristides' leg, many physicians were summoned for deliberation and a medical conference took place.[312] Various treatment-options were suggested, such as surgery and cauterisation by drugs, which suggests that all the physicians shared a professional language and agreed upon the inclusion of certain procedures within the scope of medical activity. The most conclusive proof of a lack of mutual exclusion between the various schools of health-care providers in the *Sacred Tales*, however, can be seen in the figure of Asclepiacus, the temple warden, who is described interchangeably as a temple warden and a physician.[313]

The world of the *Sacred Tales* has physicians offering medical care to the convalescents of the Asclepieion, providing them with authoritative advice with regard to the interpretation of dreams, performing medical procedures such as enemas and phlebotomies and even joining them in their journeys to undergo purges in certain divinely designated sites. For example, when Asclepius instructed Aristides to embark on a journey to bathe in an ice-cold river in the middle of winter he was accompanied by various physicians as well as by friends.[314] The only physician mentioned by name is Heracleon (otherwise unknown), who cast doubt on the ability of Aristides' body to endure the cold, but he was proven wrong and ended up acknowledging the supremacy of Asclepius' regimen, at least according to the *Sacred Tales*. In sum, the world of the *Sacred Tales* portrays three groups of health-care provider, each distinguished enough to be denoted by a generic name alone, who perceived members of the other groups as relevant and accessible when offering health-care. The existence of acknowledged health care providers and a vocabulary which described them proves that there were general criteria to guide the patient when seeking health-care and to evaluate treatment-approaches which existed prior to and independently from individual episodes of sickness. The fact that

---

310 Consulting Heracleon: Aristid. *Or.* 48.20 K; Porphyrio: Aristid. *Or.* 47.57 K; Satyrus: Aristid. *Or.* 49.8–10 K; Theodotus: Aristid. *Or.* 48.34; 50.38, 42 K.

311 Aristid. *Or.* 47.62 K.

312 Aristid. *Or.* 47.62 K.

313 Asclepiacus as a doctor: Aristid. *Or.* 49. 25 K ('Ασκληπιακὸν τὸν ἰατρὸν ἐδόκουν εἰσελθόντα ...); as a priest: Aristid. *Or.* 47. 58, 76, 48. 35 K, 49.22 (ἐπέρχεται ὁ νεωκόρος ὁ 'Ασκληπιακός ...).

314 παρέπεμπον ἡμᾶς οἱ φίλοι καὶ τῶν ἰατρῶν οἵ τε δὴ συνήθεις καὶ ἄλλοι. Aristid. *Or.* 48.20 K.

Aristides consulted physicians, gymnastic trainers, and temple wardens when he was ill is an example of how particular illness episodes were managed through communicative operations, such as labelling and explaining. Identifying the health care providers which Aristides turned to and recognizing the origin of their authority is paramount for an investigation of the health care system in Aristides' world.

Medical Praxis

Although the *Sacred Tales* bear no trace of a medical paradigm in a modern/scientific sense,[315] they do portray a clear notion of proper and improper medical conduct which is indicative of an established medical praxis and an established medical discourse. For example, when Aristides described his period in the Asclepieion (i.e. his *cathedra*)[316] he said that at this time he was almost cured and that the god prescribed him a new regimen, which he was happy to follow, but he was persuaded to follow the unwise counsel of those 'who pretending to wisdom and, seeming to have a certain cleverness in these matters, explained my dreams rather unnaturally' (οἳ σοφίας τε ἀντιποιούμενοι καί τινα ἔχειν περὶ ταῦτα δοκοῦντες δεινότητα ἀτοπώτερον τὰ ἐνύπνια ἐξηγοῦντο).[317] Aristides explicitly refers to 'the errors of my advisers' βουλὴ δὲ κακὴ νίκησεν ἑταίρων).[318] This episode firstly exemplifies the particular meaning and use of dreams in the prevailing medical discourse in the temple as communicating vital medical information, with a claimed distinction between a 'natural' and an 'unnatural' interpretation. Secondly, it shows that there are specific people who are designated as knowledgeable in the medical interpretation of dreams. Finally, the use of the Homeric term 'ill advice' (βουλὴ δὲ κακή) suggests a pre-existing discipline. One can err only if there is a correct course of action which has not been taken. In consequence, it was possible to 'know' what to do—namely how to interpret the dreams Asclepius sent.

As noted above, the *Sacred Tales* portray a community of health-care practitioners. Aristides' use of their generic names (such as 'physicians', 'gymnastic trainers' and 'temple wardens') indicates that he believed their

---

315 I follow here Kuhn's definition of a scientific paradigm as the achievements of scientists which, at least for a while, dominate a particular scientific community (cf. physicians, chemists, biologists etc.) providing both good enough solutions, as well as formulations of related problems (Kuhn, [1962] 9).

316 For a discussion of this uncommon term see pp. 109–111.

317 Aristid. *Or.* 48.72 K.

318 Aristid. *Or.* 48.72 K.

identity and professional allegiance would be familiar enough to the readers of the *Sacred Tales* to require no other identification. Another indication of the existence of a professional community of health-care providers is their use of a common professional language, which becomes clear both in their use of the terms καθάρσις, φάρμκον and their cognates, and when analysing dreams.

Purgation

The meaning and use of the term κάθαρσις[319] and its cognates in the context of health-care provides compelling evidence for the existence of an established medical practice and a professional medical language in the world of the *Sacred Tales*. It also marks those who authoritatively prescribed purgation as the designated practitioners of health-care. It will be necessary, therefore, to look into the various instances where purgation was prescribed and practised in order to establish some characteristics of the medical discourse in the *Sacred Tales*.

On January 12, 166 CE Aristides dreamt that he was walking away from the propylaea of the temple of Asclepius in Smyrna and a bull menaced him right by the 'god's ear' (κατ' αὐτὰς τὰς ἀκοὰς τοῦ θεοῦ).[320] Though the bull did nothing but bruise his right knee, Aristides was alarmed. At this point 'Theodotus took a lancet and cleansed it' (ὁ δὲ Θεόδοτος σμίλην τινὰ λαβὼν ἀνεκάθαρεν).[321] Theodotus was a Pergamene physician whom Aristides consulted during his *cathedra* on a number of occasions.[322] Both the identity of Theodotus and the medical instrument he uses indicate that cleansing/purgation equates to a medical procedure.[323] Likewise, when Aristides was in Rome in the spring of 144 CE and his health collapsed he turned to some unnamed local physicians. These physicians 'produced purges, and I was purged for two days by drinking *elaterium*'.[324] Here too the notion of purging has a strictly medical sense and it is the physicians' objective to effect it. Securing purgation appears in this episode to be an indication of the

---

319 Both 'cleansing' and 'purgation' are the English translations of the Greek term κάθαρσις and are used here as synonyms.

320 Aristid. *Or.* 47.13 K; Behr (1981–1986) vol. ii. n. 23 ad loc. suggested that the 'god's ear' was probably a building in the temple's vicinity.

321 Aristid. *Or.* 47.13 K.

322 Aristid. *Or.* 47.13, 55, 56; 48.34; 50.21, 38, 42; 51.57 K.

323 ἡ σμίλη is a lancet or a surgeon's knife. Cf. Lucian, *Ind.* 29; Poll. 4.181.

324 καὶ οἱ ἰατροὶ καθάρσεις προσήγονκαὶ πις'ν ἐλατήριον εἰς δύο ἡμέρας ἐκαθαιρόμην. Aristid. *Or.* 48.63 K.

success of the medical procedures (even if this success is only a short term one) and therefore the goal of the physicians.

Cleansing in the *Sacred Tales* also had religious connotations. For example, in the winter of 148 CE Asclepius commanded Aristides 'to do many strange things. Of what I remember, there was a race, which it was necessary to run unshod in wintertime. And again horseback riding, a most difficult matter. And I also remember some such thing. When the harbour was stormy from south-west winds and boats were being tossed about, I had to sail across to the opposite side, and having eaten honey and acorns, to vomit, and so a complete purge took place'.[325] Here a strictly medical context is absent. On the contrary, the commands in this dream resemble other testimonies of Asclepius' revelations to his worshippers such as the Roman emperor Marcus Aurelius,[326] which associate the contents of this dream, and the meaning of purgation which was associated with it, with the cult of Asclepius rather than with a medical procedure in a scientific sense.

The ambiguity between a medical semantic network and that of the cult of Asclepius in the world of the *Sacred Tales* becomes evident in the narrative of Zosimus' (Aristides' foster-father) recuperation. Zosimus fell sick late in the summer of 148 CE. Aristides asked Asclepius to save his foster-father and indeed 'Zosimus recovered beyond expectation from that disease, having been purged with barley gruel and lentils, as the god foretold to me on his behalf'.[327] Here the explanatory model of the *Sacred Tales* moves naturally from a religious semantic framework of salvation into a medical one.[328] Greek medical works often discussed the merits of various kinds of foods in medical practice, with particular reference to barley. The Hippocratic author of the treatise *On Acute Diseases* acknowledged the popularity of barley as therapeutic nourishment, which must have still been the case in Aristides' day if Galen himself chose to compose a whole treatise on the qualities of barley soup.[329] However, Graeco-Roman religions often used the term of purgation in juxtaposition with defilement in a distinctively reli-

---

325 Πολλὰ μὲν οὖν καὶ παράδοξα ἐπετάχθημεν· ὧν δὲ ἀπομνημονεύω, δρόμος τέ ἐστιν ὃν ἔδει δραμεῖν ἀνυπόδητον χειμῶνος ὥρᾳ· καὶ πάλιν ἱππασία πραγμάτων ἀπορώτατον. καί τι καὶ τοσοῦτον μέμνημαι· τοῦ γὰρ λιμένος κυμαίνοντος ἐξ ἀνέμου λιβὸς καὶ τῶν πλοίων ταραττομένων, ἔδει διαπλεύσαντα εἰς τὸ ἀντιπέρας μέλιτος καὶ δρυὸς βαλάνων φαγόντα ἐμέσαι, καὶ γίγνεται δὴ κάθαρσις ἐντελής. Aristid. *Or.* 47.65 K.

326 Cf. M.Ant. 5.8.1.

327 προῶτον μὲν ἀνίσταται παρ' ἐλπίδας ἐξ ἐκείνης τῆς νόσου ὁΖώσιμος, καθαρθείς γε διὰ πτισάνης καὶ φακῆς, προειπόντος ἐμοὶ τοῦ θεοῦ ὑπὲρ αὐτοῦ. Aristid. *Or.* 47.72 K.

328 The use of the term 'medical' here discloses my own modern perspective.

329 Hippoc. *Acut.* 6; Gal. 6.816–831 K.

gious meaning.[330] Hence the ancient reader of the *Sacred Tales* was likely to have understood Zosimus' recuperation both as a medical narrative and as a religious one. A modern student of Graeco-Roman medicine, on the other hand, reading about the recuperation of Zosimus, can see a medical discourse which has yet to distinguish its scientific notions from religious ones.

Purgation was an important aspect of the cult of Asclepius.[331] There were regular public purification ceremonies in the temple of Asclepius,[332] and the god often sends Aristides to purge.[333] Asclepius was not the only deity who instructed Aristides to perform rites of purgation though. After a revelation of Athena in a vision during the summer of 165 CE Aristides had a wash (κλύσμα) of Attic honey 'and there was a purge of my bile' (καὶ ἐγένετο κάθαρσις χολῆς).[334] Here again the narrative of the *Sacred Tales* moves with ease between the medical field and that of religion. κλύσμα was a common medical procedure and the notion of bile was one of the foundations of Greek medicine as a whole.[335] Moreover, this is not the only occurrence of the notion of bile in the *Tales*. In the winter of 148 CE, while at his ancestral estates, Aristides fell ill and members of his household ran to call for a physician. While waiting for the physician to arrive Aristides 'had an attack, and not much later I had a bowel movement of black bile' (πάλιν προσβολή τις προσῄει, καὶ μετ' οὐ πολὺ διεχώρει κάτω μέλαινα):[336] Galen himself used a cognate of the verb διαχώρειν to denote changes in bile in his treatise *On the Natural Faculties*,[337] which suggests that Galen and Aristides shared a mutual understanding as to the mechanism of the human body and the faculties of bile within it. An analysis of the meaning and the use of the term κάθαρσις thus indicates that both the gods' prescription of procedures which are essentially medical, and Aristides' understanding of their motives with terms and notions that originated in Greek medical works. The world

---

330 Cf. Parker (1983), and, concentrating on medicine, Leven (1993) 44–73.

331 Cf. Aristid. Or. 50.6 K; *I.Perg*. II.264.

332 Aristid. *Or*. 48.31 K.

333 Cf. Aristid. *Or*. 48.11, 13, 14, 28 K. Such a journey was analyzed by Rutherford (1999)133–148; I discussed this further in: Israelowich (2007) 105–108.

334 Aristid. *Or*. 48.43 K.

335 κλύσμα: Ruf. *ap*. Orib. 8.24 tit; 7.26.191; τὸ κλυσματικόν: Hippoc. *Epid*. 3.17; Ruf. *Ren. Ves.* 1.etc; ὁ κλυσμός: Ruf. *ap*. Orib. 7.26.18; κλυστέος, α, ον: Lycus. *ap. Orib*. 8.28.7; ὁ κλυστήρ: Lycus. *ap*. Orib. 8.33.3; Sor. 2.59; Gal. 10.358 K; τὸ κλυστήριον: Gal. 7.443 K; τὸ κλυστηρίδιον: Sor. 1.125.

336 Aristid. *Or*. 49.18–19 K. Keil's note here: μέλαινα] sc. χολή, e medicorum dictione.

337 τὰ μὲν διαχωρήματα μηδὲν ὅλως ἐν αὐτοῖς ἔχοντα χολῆς. Gal. *De naturalibus facultatibus*, 1.13 p. 40 K.

of the *Sacred Tales* did not draw a border-line between a medical semantic network and that of temple medicine. An analysis of the meaning and the use of notions inferring purgation yields nothing less than a map both 'for' and 'of' human behaviour within the field of health care. It reveals how a system of symbolic meanings was anchored 'in particular arrangements of social institutions and patterns of interpersonal interactions'.[338] Another example of the ambiguous meaning—either medical or religious—of the term κάθαρσις in the *Sacred Tales* is the account of the meeting between Aristides and the physician Satyrus at Pergamum in 147 CE. Satyrus was a physician of distinction. He must have been a scholar and a social peer of Aristides who calls him 'a sophist of no mean rank' (σοφιστής, ὡς ἐλέγετο, οθ' τῶν ἀγεννῶν).[339] He was also Galen's teacher while studying in Pergamum.[340] Satyrus visited Aristides when he was lying in his sickbed and in the course of their conversation Aristides told him of the 'many purges of blood I have had' (τὰς καθάρσεις τοῦ αἵματος ἤκουσεν ὅσαι γεγόνασί μοι).[341] The famous physician ordered Aristides to quit performing blood purgation, fearing it would weaken his body and threaten his life. Instead he prescribed an ointment. Aristides used the ointment, but refrained from abandoning the purgation. It is only then that the reader learns that it is Asclepius who had prescribed the purges:

> ταῦτα συνεβούλευε, κἀγὼ τὸ μὲν τοῦ αἵματος οὐκ ἔφην εἶναι κύριος οὔτε οὕτως οὔτ' ἐκείνως ποιεῖν, ἀλλ' ἕως ἂν ὁ θεὸς προστάττῃ ἀφαιρεῖν, ὑπακούσεσθαι καὶ ἑκὼν καὶ ἄκων, μᾶλλον δὲ οὐδέποτε ἄκων· τὴν δόσιν δὲ οὐκ ἔφυγον τοῦ Σατύρου, ἀλλ' ἐφύλαττον λαβών.[342]

Purgation of blood was a common medical procedure in classical medicine and Satyrus and Asclepius clearly used the same word with a reference to the same medical procedure, hence they shared a common professional language. Moreover Satyrus did not dismiss Asclepius' prescription as non-medical, or irrelevant to his own prescription. He questions the utility of phlebotomy as one physician questions a regimen another has prescribed.

338 Cf. Geertz (1973) 3–30; Kleinman (1980) 24.
339 Aristid. *Or.* 49.8 K.
340 Gal. 2.224; 19.58 K.
341 Aristid. *Or.* 49.8 K.
342 'He [i.e. Satyrus] advised these things. And as regards my blood, I said that I did not have the authority to do one thing or the other, but that while the god commanded the letting of my blood, I would obey whether willing or not, or rather never unwillingly. Still I did not ignore Satyrus' prescription, but took and kept it'. Aristid. *Or.* 49.9 K.

A study of the meaning and use of κάθαρσις in the *Sacred Tales* supports the existence of a medical discourse and demonstrates that this discourse was shared by physicians and religious healers alike. Firstly the meaning of κάθαρσις appears to have strong links with health-care activities, be these activities scientifically motivated or religiously explained by the need to avoid sin and defilement. Secondly, those who were recognised as health-care providers, both physicians and priests, often prescribed cleansing as part of their treatment. The existence of a term which designated a medical procedure and the common use of this term by recognisable health-care providers is indicative of a well-established medical discourse.

Pharmakon

The *Sacred Tales* contain many appearances of the term φάρμακον in a medical context. φάρμακον had long been a seminal notion in Graeco-Roman medicine,[343] and a study of its meaning and use in the *Sacred Tales* can place this work in the wider context of Graeco-Roman medicine.

The term φάρμακον is used in the *Sacred Tales* to mean a drug: 'I thought that it would be above all suitable to be a drug for cold' (ἐνθυμηθῆναι ὡς ἐπιτηδείως ἔχοι παντὸς μᾶλλον ψύξεως εἶναιφάρμακον).[344] But it also used to refer to a poison in other instances: 'next the prophet Corus was present and showed that there was a quick acting poison in them' (ἔπειτα παρόντα Κόρον τὸν μάντιν δεῖξαι ὅτι ἐωείη φάρμακον τῶν ἐφημέρων),[345] and 'next someone said that there was also some poison in another of the figs' (ἔπειτα φάναι τινὰ ὅτι καὶ ἐν ἄλλῳ τῳ τῶν σιτίων εἴη τοῦ φαρμάκου).[346] On most occasions the *Sacred Tales* are reluctant to give any details about the characteristics of the φάρμακον prescribed. The generic name seems to have been descriptive enough. The characteristics of the φάρμακον Asclepius prescribed Aristides during the winter of 148 CE—'there was a certain drug, whose particulars I do not remember, except that it contained salt' (ἦν δέ τι φάρμακον οὗ τὰ μὲν καθ' ἕκαστα οὐ μέμνημαι, ἁλῶν δὲ ὅτι μετεῖχεν)[347] is as detailed a description as the reader is provided with.

Though prescribing a φάρμακον had a strictly medical connotation, its prescription was not restricted to physicians. A φάρμακον could also be a cure from the god: ὁ μὲν γὰρ θεὸς προὔλεγεν ἐκ πολλοῦ δεῖν ὕδερον φύλλασε-

---

343 See above, pp. 48–49.

344 Aristid. *Or.* 47.26 K.

345 Aristid. *Or.* 47.54 K.

346 Aristid. *Or.* 47.54 K.

347 Aristid. *Or.* 47.66 K.

σθαι, καὶ ἄλλα τε ἔδωκεν ἀλειξιφάρμακα καὶ θ'ποδήματα Αἰγύπτια ('the god ... he gave me various drugs and Egyptian slippers').[348] However, there is no apparent difference in the nature of either the drug itself or in the meaning of the act of prescribing it when it was done by either a deity or human physician. For instance when physicians prescribed a φάρμακον to Aristides when he had a tumour: ἐνταῦθα οἱ μὲν ἰατροὶ πάσας φωνὰς ἠφίεσαν, οἱ μὲν τέμνειν, οἱ δὲ ἐπικάειν φαρμάκοις,[349] ('at this point the physicians cried out all sorts of things, some said surgery, some cauterisation by drugs') it seemed identical, both in its execution and intention to when the god prescribed it. Finally Asclepius prescribed a drug which dissolves the blockage and made the tumour disappear with a final application of an egg which removed all trace of the tumour.[350]

It is, however, implicit in the narrative of the *Tales* that Aristides' willingness to use the prescribed φάρμακον had much to with the identity of the medicator. While Aristides was unwilling to use the φάρμακον of the unnamed physicians when his tumour appeared, he was less reluctant to apply a φάρμακον that the famous physician Satyrus prescribed, and he never refused a φάρμακον of a deity. The identification of the φάρμακον by its medicator (cf. τὸ τοῦ Σατύρου φάρμακα)[351] suggests that personal trust was fundamental. The common terminology in the case of φάρμακα proves the existence of a social mechanism of regulating scientific activity. The implication of this social mechanism was, using Barton's terminology, that science is interwoven within a discourse of power.[352] Aristides shares with his readers his deliberations as to whether he ought to use Satyrus' φάρμακον, or instead continue with the regimen Asclepius had prescribed. Eventually Aristides used Satyrus' φάρμακον, but he explains his choice by stating that this φάρμακον of Satyrus did not contradict that of the god. The outcome, however, was rather disappointing: Satyrus' φάρμακον disagreed with Aristides.

The use of φάρμακον by physicians in the *Sacred Tales* supports the argument that Graeco-Roman physicians viewed obtaining their patients' consent to use their φάρμακα as a vote of confidence (as was noted above).[353] It also portrays the particular nature of power distribution within the

348 Aristid. *Or.* 47.61 K.
349 Aristid. *Or.* 47.63 K the same use and meaning of φάρμακον.
350 Aristid. *Or.* 47.63 K; cf. Petsalis-Diomidis (2010) 112.
351 'The drug of Satyrus' Aristid. *Or.* 49.10 K.
352 Barton (1994).
353 See above, pp. 48–49.

Graeco-Roman health care system. Aristides' decision not to follow the regimen his physicians prescribed when he had a tumour, to refuse using their φάρμακον, and to hold on to the course Asclepius had offered, demonstrates that as a patient Aristides' willingness to follow his physicians' counsel could not be taken for granted.[354] The ambiguity in the meaning of φάρμακον—it could have been taken either as a medicine or as a poison—emphasised the patient's act of faith in taking such a drug. In addition, the *Sacred Tales* often describe the φάρμακον of Aristides' physicians as ineffective. For example, while in Rome during 144 CE Aristides was treated by local physicians who implemented various medical tools in vain attempts to restore his health. In addition to chirurgical means they also used drugs: 'antidotes and various other drugs were given in vain' (φάρμακα δὲ θήρειά τε καὶ ἄλλα παντοῖα τηνάλλως ἐδίδοτο).[355] The inability of physicians to restore Aristides' health—initially in Rome, in Macedonia and Thrace and later in Smyrna—is contrasted in the *Sacred Tales* with the usefulness of Asclepius as a physician. Aristides never questioned Asclepius' prescriptions, which often included a φάρμακον. This was not the case with his human physicians. Asclepius' φάρμακα are useful; those of his human physicians are not.

The meaning and use of the term φάρμακον in the *Sacred Tales* is consistent with many other instances from the Graeco-Roman medical tradition. Both in its wide spectrum of meanings, as well as in its role as a medical procedure, the *Sacred Tales* reflect and reinforce previous Graeco-Roman medical works. The function of a φάρμακον in the relationship between patients and healers in Graeco-Roman medicine in general, and in the *Sacred Tales* in particular, demonstrates what physicians had to do in order to secure the trust of their patients. The ability of a deity to prescribe a φάρμακον shows that in some cases the physician had to excel in merit not only in comparison to his peers, but also to his gods.

Dreams

The existence of a group of well-recognised health-care providers in the world of the *Sacred Tales*, and their common use of a professional language, is also attested by their approach to dreams. All the actors taking part in the medical discourse in the *Sacred Tales*, both health-care providers and the sick themselves, shared a similar understanding of the nature of dreams. Dreams, as noted earlier in the chapter, were commonly believed to exist

354 Aristid. *Or.* 47.63 K.
355 Aristid. *Or.* 48.64 K.

autonomously and they were distinguished from the dreamer, and this was the view depicted in the *Sacred Tales*. Such a view of the dream-mechanism allows dreams to be seen as messages from a deity. In a medical context dreams can function as symptoms of physical ailments and, therefore, can be properly interpreted by those who have the appropriate knowledge, skills and expertise.

This use of dreams in medical practice depicts a spectrum of health-care practitioners broad enough to include those who practised both temple medicine and scientific medicine. In other words, the *Sacred Tales* portray a medical discourse which clearly had room for divination, mainly through dreams, in medical practice. The vast majority of the over 130 dreams that Aristides recorded in the *Sacred Tales* revolve around his medical condition. Furthermore, the explanation of these dreams was seen by both Aristides and his carers as part of the healing activities *per se*.[356] None of the physicians or members of the temple staff who assisted Aristides in interpreting his dreams voiced any fundamental disagreement about this understanding of them.[357] The physicians in the *Sacred Tales* shared Aristides' faith in Asclepius and his conception of the particular meaning and use of dreams in communication between gods and humans. For example, in February, 166 CE, while Aristides was severely ill, a physician arrived and prepared himself to help 'as much as he knew how' (ὅσα ἐπενόει) but he too was persuaded that Aristides should follow the regimen prescribed by the god 'being a sensible man' (αὐτός τε ὑπεχώρει νοῦν ἔχων).[358] This episode exemplifies that, firstly, there is no contradiction between having faith and being wise and, secondly, that physicians shared Aristides' understanding of the dream-mechanism, their divine origin and their role in providing health-care.

The Asclepieion, in this respect, provided Aristides with an environment which guided both his comprehension of his condition as well as his expectations from the treatment he underwent, as well as a medical establishment. After having one of his many god-sent dreams it was the Asclepieion which would direct Aristides towards those who were suitable to offer help. The Asclepieion also provided Aristides with a general conceptual scheme with which he could come to terms with his illness. A good example is a

356 As mentioned above, the sum of all healing activities defines the scope of the health care system, see above, pp. 40–44.
357 Cf. Aristid. *Or*. 47.57 K.
358 Aristid. *Or*. 47.57 K.

dream both Aristides and one of the two temple wardens, Philadelphus, had during the winter of 146 CE. The dream included a medical prescription: drinking wormwood diluted in vinegar and a scene from a religious festival in which a multitude of men congregated in the Sacred Theatre in the Pergamene Asclepieion, all wearing white garments and assembling before the god. The dream has it that Aristides delivered a hymn to the god during this festival.[359] The two authorities Aristides consulted on the meaning of this dream were Theodotus, a physician, whom Aristides summoned, and Asclepiacus, the temple warden, who offered Aristides help in interpreting the dream. Aristides first recounted the dream to Theodotus, who 'marvelled how divine they [i.e. the dreams] were' (ὁ δ' ἐθαύμαζε μὲν ὡς εἶχε δαιμονίως),[360] but the physician did not know how to help. Theodotus and Aristides decided to summon Asclepiacus, the temple warden, who informed Aristides that just before he called for him he was summoned by his colleague, Philadelphus, who dreamt a very similar dream about Aristides.[361] Philadelphus then joined the conversation and narrated his own dream, which concerned Aristides. Aristides tells us that 'since the dreams agreed' (ὡς δὲ συνέβαινεν)[362] he was convinced he should comply with Asclepius' prescription and Aristides went on to drink wormwood.[363] This episode demonstrates that the process of deciphering a dream and learning its 'true' meaning was a communal effort. The actual procedure of interpreting a dream was guided by a pre-existing discourse, whose authoritative representatives included both physicians and priests. The Asclepieion itself functions here as a formative and educative environment that teaches those present how to understand their dreams and trains them as participants in its discourse.

To conclude, the approach of patients and healers to dreams in the *Sacred Tales* offers another compelling proof for the existence of a vibrant medical discourse and a developed community of health-care providers during the high empire. Moreover, rather than being eccentric, Aristides' whole approach to dreams was typical of this time. The *Sacred Tales* offer a patient's personal perspective on an oneirocritical and medical tradition that dated back to the days of Homer if not earlier.[364] A very similar

359 Aristid. *Or.* 48.29–36 K.
360 Aristid. *Or.* 48.34 K.
361 Aristid. *Or.* 48.35 K.
362 Aristid. *Or.* 48.35 K.
363 Aristid. *Or.* 48.36 K.
364 See above, 'Dreams' pp. 71ff.

comprehension of dreams is found in the work of Artemidorus, Aristides' contemporary, in his treatise on dream-interpretation.[365] Though Artemidorus was mainly concerned with the ability of dreams to predict the future and his discussion of their medical traits is only marginal, it appears that the role of dreams in a medical discourse, as seen in the *Sacred Tales*, was based on a widely accepted comprehension of the dream-mechanism and the nature of the gods. The meaning and use of dreams in the *Sacred Tales* demonstrates both the existence of a medical discourse in the world of the *Sacred Tales*, as well as the deep roots of this medical discourse in traditional Greek thought.

Medical Procedures and the Physicians

The *Sacred Tales* contain many instances when health-care providers and the sick agree about the nature of medical procedures indicating a shared understanding of medical practice. For example, when Aristides returned to Smyrna from Rome in November, 144 CE, the 'physicians and gymnastic trainers assembled' (καὶ συνῆλθον οἵ τε ἰατροὶ καὶ γυμνασταὶ) to offer health-care.[366] Though they were unable to find agreement as to the cause and nature of Aristides' illness they concurred that he should be brought to the warm springs.[367] Later on, in August 165 CE, when his throat troubled him, Aristides recalls a prescription physicians usually give in such circumstances: gargling.[368] On other occasions the existence of a medical praxis in the world of the *Sacred Tales* is revealed through Aristides' descriptions of disagreements, usually between physicians and Asclepius. On more than one occasion, the god prescribes Aristides a regimen that seemed to his physicians inadequate or dangerous, hence contradicting an established medical praxis. Such are Asclepius' commands that Aristides will bathe in springs, seas and rivers in high winter and go through excessive phlebotomies, all of which met fierce objections from physicians.[369] On other occasions, the prescription of the god was in direct opposition to medical praxis. For example Asclepius prescribed Aristides a certain drug, which he should consume after dining, but the physicians disapproved because they

365 Ibid.
366 Aristid. *Or.* 48.69 K.
367 Aristid. *Or.* 48.69 K.
368 Aristid. *Or.* 51.9 K.
369 The physician Heracleon objected to Asclepius' command from the winter of 149 CE that Aristides should bathe in an icy river, predicting he will be afflicted with muscle spasms: Aristid. *Or.* 48.19–20 K.

did not believe the drug should be taken with food.[370] Aristides complied with Asclepius' regimen, which proved effective, and he used this example to demonstrate the merits of following Asclepius, a key theme of the *Sacred Tales*. However, as argued before, the *Tales* were not conceived of as a medical treatise and their usefulness to medical history is often only oblique. Nonetheless, they do provide clear evidence for the existence of general criteria which guided the health-care seeking process. This criteria evaluated treatment-approaches existing prior to and independently from individual episodes of sickness, which is one of the cornerstones of a health care system.[371] Moreover, descriptions of the management of particular illness episodes through communicative operations, such as labelling and explaining, are amply provided within the *Sacred Tales*. They demonstrate that the power structure within the realm of health care was evident to the sick, such as Aristides, and was, to a large extent, explained to them by the various health care providers themselves.

The most obvious example, however, of an established medical praxis which relied on a professional language can be seen in the context of dream-interpretation. It is noteworthy that even though Aristides viewed himself as having direct relations with Asclepius he often had to rely on others for interpreting his dreams. At times Asclepius confirmed his diagnosis of Aristides and prescribed him a regimen by communicating with others, such as Theodotus, Philadelphus and Asclepiacus who were all medical authorities.[372] In his capacity as a temple warden Asclepiacus regularly helped Aristides to interpret his dreams and to find the exact remedy the god prescribed. For example, during the summer of 148 CE Aristides had difficulties in breathing and the god prescribed 'a royal ointment' (χρῖμα ἔφη βασιλικὸν εἶναι).[373] Aristides did not know what a royal ointment meant, but the temple warden easily directed him towards an ointment which lay at the feet of Hygieia.[374] This example of a successful interpretation of a dream provides another indication of the formative role of society in general, and of the environment of the Asclepieion in particular, in shaping Aristides' experiences. The narrative of the *Sacred Tales* can

---

370 Aristid. *Or*. 49.27 K.

371 Cf. Kleinman (1980) 71–72.

372 Theodotus: Aristid. *Or*. 48.34, 50.42 K; Philadephus: Aristid. *Or*. 48.31–35 K; Asclepiacus: Aristid. *Or*. 48.31–35; 49.14 K. There is also a mentioning of an unnamed Macedonian: Aristid. *Or*. 50.42 K.

373 Aristid. *Or*. 49.21 K.

374 Aristid. *Or*. 49.22 K.

therefore offer evidence for the existence of a medical establishment, language and praxis in the second century CE.

Having established the existence of a discernable conceptual scheme which directed and regulated health-care within the world of the *Sacred Tales*, it is possible to carry this argument further and characterise some of its key attributes, namely the synergy between temple medicine and health-care which had a more scientific approach. During Aristides' *cathedra* Asclepius commanded him to spend time on songs and lyric verse, and to relax and maintain a chorus of boys.[375] This regimen was so effective that whenever Aristides 'happened to choke, if my throat were suddenly constricted, or my stomach became disordered, or whenever I had some other troublesome attack, the physician Theodotus, being in attendance and remembering my dreams, used to order the boys to sing some of my lyric verse. And while they were singing, there arose unnoticed a feeling of comfort, and sometimes everything which pained me went completely away'.[376] It is left to the reader to decide which aspect of this treatment was so effective and why. It could be the boys' singing, the content of Aristides' lyric verse or the mere fact that it was Asclepius' regimen. Whatever the answer, the physician supported Aristides' religious propensity and provided his choice with the sanction of the medical establishment. No marked boundary between religious healing and scientific medicine is revealed.

The Physicians in the Sacred Tales

The constant need of physicians to compete for their patients' trust raises a more general question about the identity of the physicians, their relationship with their patients and about the physician as an artisan in the world of the *Sacred Tales*. The place of physicians in society, according to the *Sacred Tales*, ranged from the heights of a figure such as Satyrus, who appears to be Aristides' peer in his social status, through Theodotus, Heracleon and Porphyrio who are mentioned by name, down to the Smyrnean physicians who cared for Aristides during the great plague and then replaced his domestic servants after they died from the plague.[377]

---

375 Aristid. *Or.* 50.38 K.

376 καὶ ὁπότε ἢ πνίγεσθαι συμβαίνοι, τοῦ τραχήλου ταθέντος ἐξαίφνης ἢ τοῦ στομάχου καταστάντος εἰς ἀπορίας, ἤ τις ἄλλη γένοιτο ἄπορος προσβολή, παρὼν ἂν Θεόδοτος ὁ ἰατρὸς καὶ μεμνημένος τῶν ἐνυπνίων ἐκέλευε τοὺς παῖδας ᾄδειν τῶν μελῶν, καὶ μεταξὺ ᾀδόντων λάθρα τις ἐγίγνετο ῥᾳστώνη, ἔστι δ' ὅτε καὶ παντελῶς ἀπῄει πᾶν τὸ λυποῦν. Aristid. *Or.* 50.38 K.

377 Aristid. *Or.* 48.37–39 K.

Similarly, the nature of medical authority itself varied from being the result of common sense, practice and life-experience to medicine as a discipline, which is based on scholarship and learning. The *Sacred Tales* have on the one hand Zosimus, Aristides' servant and foster-father, who, during the winter of 148 CE, travelled by foot a distance of forty stades to visit another sick servant of Aristides and to offer him medical help 'for he was also skilled in medicine' (ἦν γὰρ δὴ καὶ τὴν τέχνην ἀγαθὸς τὴν ἰατρικήν).[378] On the other hand we have Satyrus, whom Aristides describes as a scholar and whose discernable medical learning is still reflected in the work of Galen, his student.[379] Nonetheless it is notable that within the *Sacred Tales* both Zosimus and Satyrus are described as skilled in medicine. Their common identity was based on the fact they were both seeking their patient's trust, and hence their patronage, in return for offering treatment and cure.

This section has examined medical practice in the Graeco-Roman world and the attitude of society towards its sick; it has asked whether there was a discernible medical discourse; and has inquired into the identity of the physicians in the world of the *Sacred Tales*. The picture which has emerged is one in which the sick formed an active part of society, rather than being a community of outcasts excluded from its social life. The existence of a medical discourse has been revealed through the identification of a particular group of health-care providers (physicians, gymnastic trainers and the priests in the Asclepieion), who shared a common professional language and recognised similar actions as medical procedures. Acquaintance with this discourse and with the meaning and use of some of its key notions, such as κάθαρσις, φάρμακον and the interpretation of dreams allows a clearer description and a deeper understanding of the world of the *Sacred Tales* by establishing more accurate taxonomies and placing medicine in its due context. The information which the *Sacred Tales* hold about the identity of individual physicians, such as personal names, social standing and quality of education, contributes to our acquaintance with this profession in the Graeco-Roman world. It portrays physicians as craftsmen with a social background which varied from the heights of the educated elite of Pergamum (Satyrus) to anonymous physicians who shared the social status of Aristides' domestic servants. Finally, the particular manner in which the medical discourse in the *Sacred Tales* was anchored to broader social institutions, notably

---

[378] Aristid. *Or.* 47.75 K.

[379] Satyrus as a scholar: Aristid. *Or.* 49.8–10K; Gal. 2.224; 19.58 K.

religion, adds to this contextualisation of ancient medicine. Mythology, theology and cosmology supplemented medicine, much of whose explanatory model was provided by patterns of thought which were borrowed from philosophy and science. Moreover, social and institutionalised forms of religious cult which were practised in the Asclepieia, amongst other places, regulated medical praxis and provided much of the social setting in which the *Sacred Tales* took place. This description, which agrees with more general studies, further reveals the contribution the *Sacred Tales* can make to the history of ancient medicine.

3. Towards a Medical History of Aelius Aristides

A medical history of Aristides is both a history of his physiology, i.e. a record and classification of his pathologies, and a history of the ideas and notions with which Aristides comprehended his medical condition and conceptualised his illness. Aristides' description of his medical condition enables us to compose a list of his symptoms according to their chronological appearance.[380] These can be divided into two groups: from 144 CE to 149 CE they are mostly respiratory; from 166 CE to 171 CE they are intestinal, and, according to one modern view, the after-effects of smallpox.[381] One must be cautious, however, when trying to form a medical diagnosis from these symptoms. Firstly, as Behr has concluded: 'it is undeniable that Aristides suffered many real diseases. But his stamina, sudden recoveries, euphoria, and depressions also point to many psychosomatic symptoms'.[382] Secondly,

380 On the physical symptoms see Behr (1968) 164–165; Schröder (1986) 11–12.

381 Behr (1968) 164–168. Identification of the great plague of 165 CE as smallpox is still a cause for dispute amongst scholars. Gilliam (1961); R.J. & M.L. Littman (1973) and Nutton (2000) 965 suggested the plague was smallpox, but Birley (2000) 168 did not exclude examthematous typhus and bubonic plague as possibilities.

382 Behr (1968) 163. Aristides' autobiographical description does, however, receive the unexpected support of the authoritative physician Galen, who remarked that Aristides had a weak body and a strong soul. Galen thought Aristides was consumptive. Preserved in the Arabic translation of Galen's *Commentary on Plato's Timaeus*. See Schröder *CMG*, Suppl. 1. 1934, p. 33. Also quoted by Behr (1968) 162. There is no proof, however, that the famous Pergamene physician had inspected Aristides in person, or even that the two men had met. Bowersock (1969) 60–61, assumed such an encounter was highly plausible; Behr (1968) 162–163, doubts it. The diagnosis could have easily reached Galen from one of his teachers, probably Satyrus of Smyrna who personally inspected Aristides. Aristid. *Or.* 49.8 K. Satyrus was a Greek physician who worked in the second century CE and was a student of Quintus (Gal. 2.217 K) and a teacher of Galen when in Pergamum (Gal. 2.224; 19.58 K). His work rested on Quintus' interpretation of the Hippocratic Corpus with a particular interest in anatomy and pharmacology. Nutton *s.v.* Satyrus in *DNP*.

Petsalis-Diomidis rightfully warned the reader against an 'over-realistic' reading of the *Sacred Tales*.[383] Such a reading, she argued, assumes that Aristides' 'journal' offers the reader a clear and intimate picture of the author, devoid of the artifice of self-presentation.[384] Following Pearcy's study of the text, Petsalis-Diomidis explained Aristides' concern with the credibility of the *Sacred Tales* among the wider audience as a rhetorical means rather than a genuine attempt at providing a realistic portrayal of the experience of an ill individual.[385] Likewise, Petsalis-Diomidis was inclined to read Aristides' exhortation to his readers who wanted to know exactly the things which happened to him to consult the parchments and the dreams themselves—where they could also find Asclepius's cures of various sorts—as an elaborate rhetorical device.[386] Questioning the very existence of these documents, let alone their availability to the reader, she argued that all reference to them was likely aimed at achieving a rhetorical goal.[387] As someone who is not a trained physician, I do not attempt the task of writing a history of Aristides' physiology and pathologies in a modern/scientific fashion; an enterprise I doubt is feasible with the evidence available. However, it is possible to undertake a contextual history of Aristides' thoughts about his medical condition and this will form the next section of this part.

Any endeavour to write such a medical history of Aristides inevitably encounters some methodological difficulties. At the beginning of the first *Sacred Tale* Aristides writes that this work is a record of the benevolence of god, a claim he reiterates at the opening of the second *Sacred Tale*.[388] Hence, the *Sacred Tales* are not a medical history; they are a eulogy to a gracious deity, and like his orations they are λόγοι.[389] Tellingly, Aristides chose not to follow a chronological narrative. Equally tantalising is the twofold dialogue of the *Sacred Tales*. The first is the dialogue between Aristides' present self and his past self—Aristides did not compose the

383 Petsalis-Diomidis (2010) 122.

384 Petsalis-Diomidis (2010) 123.

385 Aristid. *Or.* 47.62–68; 48.20 K; Pearcy (1988); Petsalis-Diomidis (2010) 130.

386 Aristid. *Or.* 48.8 K.

387 Petsalis-Diomidis (2010) 128; cf. Pearcy (1988) *passim.*

388 Aristid. *Or.* 47.3; 48.2–3K. However, Pearcy (1988) Holmes (2008); and Petsalis-Diomidis (2010) all emphasised the rhetorical nature of the *Sacred Tales* which led them to see in this text an expression of a self-conscious *pepaideumenos* whose claims about the composition of the text cannot be accepted at face value.

389 Cf. Pearcy (1988), and Petsalis-Diomidis (2010) 122–132.

Tales until sometime after the event when he finally decided to yield to requests of friends and gods to write them.[390] The second dialogue is that of the author with his prospective audience. This first dialogue poses the methodological difficulties of evaluating a work written with hindsight. The second poses, perhaps, even greater challenges because the intention of Aristides in writing the *Sacred Tales*, and the identity of his prospective readers, must also be taken into account.

A 'medical history' of Aristides therefore aims to achieve three goals: (i) a chronological arrangement of the various pieces of evidence provided by the *Sacred Tales* and other sources about Aristides' illness and the measures he took to confront it; (ii) an understanding of Aristides' own notions of disease, medicine and health care; and (iii) an examination of how Aristides constructed his account of being ill, and what were his intentions in doing so. Such a medical history will not be limited to either a literal understanding of the text or to one which assumes a hidden intention since it places the text as its object rather than as a means for reaching Aristides the person. To address these principal aims a number of more specific questions will also be considered, such as whether the Aristides of the *Sacred Tales* saw any causal and mechanistic relationship between either disease and (its) symptoms or between medical procedures and recuperation; whether Aristides depicted a dichotomy between scientific medicine and temple medicine; on what grounds Aristides chose one treatment option over another; and finally how familiar he was with the anatomy of the human body.

The section is divided into three parts. The first discusses Aristides' account of falling ill. Secondly, the main body of the section will examine Aristides' relationship with Asclepius, his attitudes towards physicians and priests, and his understanding of his illness. The final part will place Aristides' experiences in the wider social context of the time, and will look at how Aristides' health was affected by the well-being of the empire as a whole.

Falling Ill

Aristides fell sick for the first time when travelling in Egypt after the death of his father. His illness interrupted his travels and Aristides left Egypt via Alexandria and returned to Smyrna in 142 CE. However, while still in Egypt, Aristides approached a healing deity, Sarapis. This deity was also

390 Aristid. *Or.* 48.2–3 K and see chapter 1 above.

worshipped in Smyrna and on his return to the city, probably on the eve of the civic festival on April 25 in honour of this god or Zeus Sarapis, Aristides delivered his speech *To Sarapis*.[391] Aristides' health must have then stabilised and there is no report (in the *Sacred Tales* or elsewhere) of any physical inconvenience until the time when, a couple of years later in January 144 CE, Aristides embarked on a journey to Rome seeking the fame and glory the city could offer orators of exceptional skill. The last section of the journey took him by land over the Via Egnatia, but the harsh weather conditions affected Aristides' fragile health and by the time he arrived at Hellespont, long before setting foot on the Via Egnatia, his ears began to trouble him immensely and his general health deteriorated. Aristides felt that his teeth were about to fall out and 'I was in such a despair regarding my teeth, that I held out my hands in readiness, in expectation of catching them at any moment' (καὶ τοῦτο μὲν περὶ τῶν ὀδόντων ἐν παντὶ κατέστην, ὥσθ' ὑπεῖχον τὰς χεῖρας, ὡς ἀεὶ δεξόμενος).[392] In addition, Aristides could not consume anything but milk. A shortness of breath and strong fevers compounded his condition and by the time he reached Edessa in Macedonia his health collapsed.[393] He eventually gathered his strength and carried on to Rome, arriving in the city one hundred days after leaving.[394]

In Rome Aristides' intestines swelled and he reports that he suffered from horrible shivers, which ran all through his body. He turned to local physicians who offered no more than a short term solution of purging his body, using therapeutic methods which were both unpleasant and of little use. Aristides was instructed to drink *elaterium*, a medicinal drink based on cucumber, until the expected result of bloody discharge occurred.[395] Soon afterwards Aristides was struck by a fever which brought him to the edge of death. The doctors in Rome made an incision, from his chest to his bladder:

> καὶ τέλος οἱ ἰατροὶ κατέτεμνον ἐκ τοῦ στήθους ἀρξάμενοι πάντα ἑξῆς ἄχρι πρὸς τὴν κύστιν κάτω· καὶ ὡς ἀνθήψαντο αἱ σικύαι, παντάπασι τὸ πνεῦμα ἀπελήφθη,

391 Behr (1968) 21.
392 Aristid. *Or*. 48. 62 K.
393 Ibid.
394 Ibid.
395 'And the doctors produced purges, and I was purged for two days by drinking elaterium' (καὶ οἱ ἰατροὶ καθάρσεις προσῆγον καὶ πιὼν ἐλατήριον εἰς δύο ἡμέρας ἐκαθαιρόμην) Aristid. *Or*. 48. 63 K.

> καὶ διῆλθεν ὀδύνη ναρκώδης καὶ ἄπορος φέρειν, καὶ πάντα αἵματι ἐπέφυρτο καὶ γίγνομαι ὑπέρινος.[396]
>
> And for that the physicians began cutting me, starting from the chest and going in order all the way down to the bladder. And when the cupping instruments were applied, my breathing was completely stopped, and a pain, numbing and impossible to bear, passed through me and everything was smeared with blood, and I was excessively purged.

By this time Aristides could not perform the simplest daily functions without going through extreme agony and by the autumn of 144 CE he returned home.[397]

The return journey to Smyrna in October 144 CE was almost too difficult for Aristides to bear and he reports that he 'contracted by ill-luck many varied ailments from constant sickness and stormy weather which I experienced while coming back through Thrace and Macedonia' (πολλὰ καὶ παντοῖα συνειλοχὼς τῷ σώματι ἀπὸ τῶν συνεχῶν καμάτων τε καὶ χειμώνων, οἷς ἐχρησάμην απιὼν διὰ Θρᾴκης καὶ Μακεδονίας).[398] The physicians that an anguished Aristides consulted while travelling through Thrace and Macedonia were unable to assist him. Indeed they could not even identify the nature of his disease or come up with an accurate prognosis.[399] Aristides complained of a constriction in his throat when he breathed, which was accompanied by fits of shivering.[400] Arriving back in Smyrna in November 144 CE Aristides consulted doctors and gymnastic trainers as to his medical condition, but neither group could recognise what Aristides described as the 'complex nature of my disease'.[401] The bewildered Aristides took the only advice he was given and travelled to Pergamum around December 144 CE to recline in its warm springs.[402] There he spent a long period of over a year which he entitled his 'period of inactivity' (*cathedra*).

---

396 Aristid. *Or.* 48. 63 K.

397 Aristid. *Or.* 48. 63 K.

398 Aristid. *Or.* 48. 5 K.

399 Aristides himself never used this term.

400 Aristid. *Or.* 48. 5–7 K.

401 οἵ τε ἰατροὶ καὶ γυμνασταὶ καὶ οὔτε βοηθεῖν εἶχον οὔτε ἐγνώριζον τὴν ποικιλίαν τῆς νόσου. Aristid. *Or.* 48. 69 K. ('Physicians and gymnastic trainers had neither remedy nor did they understand the complexity of my disease').

402 Convalescing in hot springs was a common practice in the Graeco-Roman world. Cf. Croon (1967); Jackson (1990): Jackson (1992); Ginouvès (1994). Boudon (1994) is an interesting study of the role of water in the prescriptions of Asclepius, according to Galen and Aristides, and Jones (1991) looked into Aristides' characterisation of the water in Pergamum.

Aristides' choice of describing his period in Pergamum with the word *cathedra* is an interesting one.[403] Although Antyllus[404] and Soranus,[405] two Greek authors writing on medicine who were contemporaries of Aristides, used this term in a medical context,[406] the term *cathedra* was not used exclusively in medical discourse. In fact, another common usage of this term in the Greek world of the second century was to designate the chair of a teacher or a paid position of a professional scholar, usually in the fields of rhetoric and philosophy.[407] Aristides arrived in Pergamum soon after he was forced to abandon his aspirations of gaining fame and glory as an orator in Rome. In the Asclepieion he resumed his engagement in rhetoric and his pursuit of a career as an orator and writer. The choice of this particular word might suggest that Aristides saw his time in Pergamum as an essential phase in his professional development.[408] His choice of the word *cathedra* to describe this time spent at the Pergamene Asclepieion might also explain why Aristides attributed his professional success to Asclepius. However, Aristides' description of this period of convalescing in the temple as *cathedra* might have been an implicit message to his readers, which placed his period of convalescing within the context of his career as a rhetor. The publication of the *Sacred Tales* makes a strong case for such an argument. The fact that the *Tales* were written to be publicly read shifts the explanation of their *raison d'être* and meaning.[409] Rather than taking

403 ἐπὶ τὴν ἐν Περγάμῳ καθέδραν ἤλθομεν. Aristid. *Or*. 48. 70 K; ἐπὶ τῆς ἐν Περγάμῳ καθέδρας. Aristid. *Or*. 49. 44 K.

404 Antyllus was a Greek physician and surgeon who lived and worked after Antigenes (late first century CE) and before Oribasius (mid-fourth century CE) and wrote about physical exercise and the various kinds of sports such as swimming, skipping, and weightlifting. Nutton *s.v.* Antyllus in *DNP* and Grant (1960). On the meaning of the term in this context cf. Petsalis-Diomidis (2010) 113.

405 Not much is now known of the life and career of Soranus of Ephesus (the best account of his life and work is Hanson and Green [1996]). From the *Suda* we learn that he was born in Ephesus and that he lived in Rome during the reign of Trajan and Hadrian. Soranus was a prolific author who wrote on various topics from grammar and etymologies to highly specialised medical topics. He also composed a number of biographies of earlier physicians, notably a *Life of Hippocrates According to Soranus*. Soranus was an erudite physician and his *Acute and Chronic Diseases* record a wide range of opinions of past medical authorities. His most important work, however, is his *Gynaecology*. Nutton (2004) 195–197.

406 Antyll. *Ap. Orib*. 9.14.6 Antyllus uses this term in a discussion of the medical qualities of beds; Sor. 1.27 Soranus, in his gynaecology, uses this term in reference to menstruation.

407 Cf. *SIG* 845 [Eleusis iii CE].

408 Cf. Cox Miller: 'This choice of name suggests that Aristides found his profession—his professing voice—not in spite of his illness that had brought him to Asclepius, but *in* it'; Cox Miller (1994) 189.

409 See 'motives for composition', above, pp. 19–23.

them as a record of Aristides' private thoughts and feelings it is necessary to see them as a message of a skilled orator to his prospective audience. Aristides' claim that it was Asclepius himself who ordered him to resume literary activity and then took an active role in Aristides' rhetorical training while at his temple, serves two purposes: it depicts Aristides' vocation as a religious calling, and it recruits a divine authority such as Asclepius to vouch for the quality of Aristides' rhetorical and scholarly work.

If indeed Aristides had a hidden agenda in writing the *Sacred Tales*, namely to glorify himself as an orator by suggesting that Asclepius was his literary patron, a history of his illness provided him with the powerful tool of a aretalogical narrative. From an initial bewilderment and helplessness when first falling ill and seeking medical help, Aristides could only find a cure by appealing to Asclepius. His career seemed to have followed a very similar path; the early promise which first encouraged Aristides to seek success as an orator in Rome was not enough. His first attempt was doomed to failure. Only after spending time in the proximity of Asclepius and benefiting from his encouragement and guidance did Aristides manage to perfect his skills and gain professional success.

Aristides had no difficulty resuming literary activity in the Asclepieion.[410] The social fabric of those present in the temple included some keen supporters of sophistic studies, both Greeks and Romans. Moreover, many of the protagonists of Philostratus' *Lives of the Greek Sophists* resided in or visited the city of Pergamum, one of the cultural and scholarly centres of the period.[411] This cultural renaissance of the Greek world in general and of Pergamum in particular, was supported by a well-disposed and philhellenic Roman government. Hadrian's remodelling of the Pergamene Asclepieion with the introduction of new buildings meant that the temple assumed the function that Hadrian had also, it is argued, assigned to the library he founded in Athens; the Pergamene Asclepieion became a centre of learning.[412] During Aristides' lifetime it was a place of congregation for

410 Behr noted that 'Aristides' social position, his earlier studies with Polemo and possibly with Aristocles, gave him an entrée to the foremost members of Pergamene society, many of whom were connected with the temple, and also quickly brought him into contact with very prominent Greeks and Romans, such as the consul Sabinus, who were convalescing there at the time ... They lived in considerable harmony, devoted to the exercises of their literary and intellectual interests, the discussion of their ailments, and the interpretation of their dreams'; Behr (1968) 42.

411 Bowersock (1969) 17–30.

412 For Hardian's visit to the temple see Le Glay (1976); on the temple see Petsalis-Diomidis (2010) chaps. 4, 5, and *passim*.

intellectuals, politicians, philosophers and writers.[413] Thus being sick, convalescing in an Asclepieion, confiding in Asclepius and following the treatment options his cult offered, were all part of social life in Asia Minor, or at least for some people in that part of the province of Asia, during the high empire.[414]

It is relevant that Aristides composed the *Tales* with hindsight of his medical history. When Aristides describes his moments of falling ill, arriving in the Asclepieion and hovering between life and death, he does so with the reassurance that only a positive outcome can provide. In a similar fashion, his general statements about his illness are the result of his own dialogue with his memories and his written records of symptoms, dreams and remedies. In this respect, the expression 'the complex nature of my disease'[415] is revealing of Aristides' persistent attempts to conceptualise his disease, and this was in turn reflected in his relationships with health-care providers and his understanding of the existing medical discourse.[416] However, these should not be viewed as Aristides' thoughts contemporaneous with the events, but rather as a result of life-long reflections and a scheme adopted in the *Sacred Tales* as a whole. A further important note is that even when compiling the *Sacred Tales* Aristides hardly ever makes a clear distinction between his illness and symptoms. He never explicitly discusses relations of cause and effect (in a mechanical sense) regarding his clinical condition and the phenomena or symptoms that resulted from it. The same absence of aetiology exists in Aristides' depictions of the treatment options offered to him, except perhaps the surgical ones.[417] None of the 130 dreams recorded in the *Sacred Tales* disclose the clinical logic of the god's prescriptions and this is probably because Aristides never sought this kind of explanation.

---

413 Hoffmann (1998) 57. Cf. Philostr. *VS* 535 (Polemo), 611 (Hermocrates).

414 Admittedly the testimony Aristides left in the *Sacred Tales* captures a reality and a form of life to which only a selected few members of the privileged members of the upper classes had access. One might recall Syme's remark here that any history is a history of its ruling classes; Syme (1939) 7. Another approach could explain the partial picture of Graeco-Roman society which we have by the nature of the evidence, not forgetting to mention that it was only the members of the upper classes who left written literary testimonies.

415 τὴν ποικιλίαν τῆς νόσου Aristid. *Or.* 48. 69 K.

416 For an analysis of the medical discourse in the *Sacred Tales* see the section 'The sick, medicine and physicians in Graeco-Roman society' above.

417 Cf. Aristid. *Or.* 47. 6–68 K.

Aristides and Asclepius

It was around December 144 CE while convalescing in the warm springs of Pergamum that Asclepius, the god of medicine, first revealed himself to Aristides and instructed him to go unshod.[418] After this first revelation Asclepius summoned Aristides to his temple in Pergamum where the god revealed himself to Zosimus, Aristides' foster-father, on Aristides' first night of incubation.[419] In addition to a general regimen, Asclepius also prescribed Aristides remedies: a sap of balsam to be used while bathing and going from the warm water to the cold. Next there was soap mixed with raisins and other things, as well as many other medicines that Aristides does not, unfortunately, list.[420]

According to the *Sacred Tales*, Aristides did not turn to Asclepius as an alternative to medicine, but rather because he thought the god was a better physician. In the opening paragraph of the first *Sacred Tale* Aristides declares that he has 'decided to submit to the god, as to a doctor and to do in silence whatever he wishes' (ὥσπερ ἰατρῷ τῷ θεῷ σιγῇ ποιεῖν).[421] During Aristides' first night of incubation the god functioned as a physician offering medicine: μετὰ δὲ ταῦτα ἐδίδου τὰ ἰάματα αὐτῷ μοι, ὧν πρῶτον ἦν, ὡς ἔγωγε μέμνημαι.[422] The dual role of Asclepius, both as a physician as well as a deity, must have been reassuring for Aristides and he certainly gained encouragement and confidence from his devotion to the god. At one time, when Aristides learned in a dream that he was fated to die in two days 'and that this was inevitable' (καὶ ταῦτα ἀναγκαίως ἔχειν)[423] the god saved him. In his dream Aristides found heartening messages from Asclepius: 'I dreamt that if I was in god's hands then there was hope' (ταῦτά τε οὕτως ἐδόκουν διαλέγεσθαι καὶ τυγχάνειν ἀκηκοὼς ὡς εἰ γενοίμην ἐν χερσὶ τοῦ θεοῦ, ἐλπίδες εἶεν).[424] On another occasion the message in the dream was that Aristides was cured.[425]

Aristides' description of his illness reveals two authorities distinguished in handling sickness—human and divine—both competing for their patient's trust. Aristides himself was conscious of this dichotomy and he

---

418 Aristid. *Or.* 48. 7 K.
419 Aristid. *Or.* 48. 8 K.
420 Aristid. *Or.* 48. 10 K.
421 Aristid. *Or.* 47. 4 K.
422 'After this he gave to me myself medicines, of which the first was, as far as I remember ...'. Aristid. *Or.* 48. 10 K.
423 Aristid. *Or.* 48. 26 K.
424 Aristid. *Or.* 47. 42 K.
425 Aristid. *Or.* 49. 5 K.

discussed the associated tension in a speech he composed during his *cathedra* in Pergamum, entitled *In Defence of Oratory*.[426] In the speech Aristides explicitly says that: 'truly just as the seers, initiated into the service of the gods who have given their name to their speciality, I have knowledge from the gods themselves. Through their aid, contrary to the likelihood of the circumstances, I am alive, having escaped at different times through various kinds of consolation and advice on the part of the god [i.e. Asclepius] from things which no doctor knew what to call, to say nothing of cure, nor had seen befall human nature'.[427] Aristides turned to the doctors when he first became sick because he wanted help in reformulating his illness, which was the sum of his physical symptoms, into a disease.[428] Disease is an abstract notion that explains certain symptoms and pathologies and is deduced by those in a society designated as capable of doing so.[429] Aristides sought an explanatory model which could tell him what was wrong with him and help him get better.[430] After his physicians were unable to provide this, Aristides turned to Asclepius. Temple medicine, though unlikely to have provided better medical treatment *per se*, offered the support and reassurance which physicians could not. Aristides' choice of Asclepius was not exclusive, however, and he did not think it needed to be. He continued to consult physicians on various occasions.

The world of the *Sacred Tales* does not present the commands of physicians and the god's exhortations as mutually exclusive sets. Neither Aristides nor his physicians drew such a dichotomy.[431] Aristides turned regularly

---

[426] Aristid. *Or.* 2. 35–36 L-B.

[427] ἀλλ' ὡς ἀληθῶς ὥσπερ οἱ θεομάντεις οἱ τοῖς τῶν πραγμάτων ἐπωνύμοις τετελεσμένοι παρ' αὐτῶν τῶν θεῶν ἔχω τὸ μάθημα, ὑφ' ὧν ἃ μηδεὶς ἰατρῶν μήτε οἶδεν ὅ τι χρὴ προσειπεῖν, οὐχ ὅπως ἰάσασθαι, μήτ' εἶδεν ἐν ἀνθρώπου φύσει συμβάντα, ἄλλοτ' ἄλλαις παραμυθίαις τε καὶ συμβουλαῖς ἐκ τοῦ θεοῦ διαφεύγων ζῶ παρὰ πᾶν τὸ ἐκ τῶν παρόντων εἰκός. Aristid. *Or.* 2. 67 L-B.

[428] Cf. Kleinman (1980) 71–72; Nijhuis (1995).

[429] As said before (in the section 'Medical knowledge and practice'), this is a prerequisite of any kind of scientific act, let alone medical diagnosis. Kuhn (1962) 9; Kleinman, (1980).

[430] One of the things a scientific community gains by establishing a paradigm is a formulation of a category of problems that can be solved. After such a paradigm is established, all other problems (namely those without a solution) are labelled as irrelevant or metaphysical. Kuhn (1962) 39. Kuhn defines 'normal science' as that which exists within such a paradigm (p. 9). Normal science produces three types of literature: (i) the establishment of important tasks for this particular branch of science. (ii) a literature which describes the compliance between theory and practice, and (iii) literature that discusses the improvement of the theory.

[431] This was no exception. Cf. Galen who refers to Asclepius as physicians' 'ancestral god' and Sextus Empiricus who refers to Asclepius as 'the founder of our [i.e. physicians] science. Gal. *De Sanitate Tuenda*, 1.8.20 K; Sext. Emp. *Math.* 1.260.

to physicians after Asclepius sent him a message either for consultation or just to explain his acts. His physicians do not seem to have found fault with this habit of Aristides. According to the *Sacred Tales*, they accepted the medical validity of his dreams and the rationale of his behaviour.[432] For instance, after a night of incubation[433] at the temple of Asclepius in Pergamum, and having received a dream from the god, Aristides summoned a physician for consultation.[434] Thus physicians did not reject temple medicine, and even more importantly the two shared a common professional language. In another dream Asclepius ordered royal ointment to be applied and Asclepiacus, the temple warden in the temple of Asclepius in Pergamum, interpreted the dream easily and provided the prescribed ointment.[435]

The position of Asclepiacus is most interesting here because Aristides describes him at times as a physician and on other occasions as a priest of Asclepius.[436] The duality of Asclepiacus captures much of the experience of Aristides in the Asclepieion as a whole. The temple warden provided the patient Aristides with lodging (Aristides resided with him during his stay in Pergamum),[437] but also with interpretations of his dreams, which are at times religious (*Or.* 49.14, 22–24 K), and at other times medical (*Or.* 48. 35 K). The significant role that Asclepiacus played in Aristides' life is attested by his frequent presence in his dreams (cf. *Or.* 47. 57, 76 K).

Aristides' willingness to follow divine prescriptions did not waver even when extreme surgical measures were instructed. In one incident Asclepius had Aristides draw blood from his elbow 'and he [i.e. the god] added, as far as I remember, one hundred and twenty litra.'[438] It is noteworthy that drawing blood from a patient was a common medical procedure in the ancient

432 Ταῦτα δὴ ἐφάνθη τὰ ὀνείρατα, ἰατροῦ τε ἥκοντος καὶ παρεσκευασμένου βοηθεῖν ὅσα ἐπενόει. ὡς δὲ ἤκουσε τῶν ὀνειράτων, αὐτός τε ὑπεχώρει νοῦν ἔχων τῷ θεῷ καὶ ἡμεῖς ἐγνωρίζομεν τὸν ἀληθινὸν καὶ προσήκοντα ἡμῖν ἰατρὸν, καὶ ἐποιοῦμεν ἃ ἐπέταξε. Aristid. *Or.* 47. 57 K.

433 Incubation was a key theme in the cult of Asclepius and Aristides went through it on various occasions e.g. Aristid. *Or.* 49. 7–8 K.

434 Aristid. *Or.* 48. 34 K.

435 Aristid. *Or.* 49. 21–23 K, and see discussion on pp. 101–103 above.

436 Asclepiacus as a doctor: Aristid. *Or.* 49. 21–23 K; as a priest: Aristid. *Or.* 47. 58, 76, 48. 35 K.

437 Aristid. *Or.* 48.35, 46–47 K.

438 πρῶτον μὲν οὖν ἐπέταξεν αἷμα ἀφελεῖν ἀπ' ἀγκῶνος καὶ προσέθηκεν, ὅσα ἐγὼ μέμνημαι, λίτριας εἴκουσι καὶ ἑκατόν. Aristid. *Or.* 48. 47 K. Aristides could not have drawn so much blood. The Greek *litra* was used as a weight measure equivalent to twelve ounces, or a pound. Even without knowing that the human body contains between four and five litters of blood, Aristides and those around him could not have believed that such a measure of blood, which is close to his entire weight, could have been drawn from him.

world.[439] Aristides consulted the meaning of this dream with the temple staff, who all contributed from their experience and knowledge. Aristides' choice to consult the meaning of his dreams can be seen as a concrete example of the health care system in operation. More specifically, it is an example of how society guided the sick when seeking health care and evaluating treatment-approaches; of how an illness episode was being managed; and of the healing activities themselves. The amount drawn was large and the 'temple wardens, being of such years, confessed that they knew of no one at all who had been operated on so much, except Ischyron, and that his case was among the strange ones, but even so mine surpassed it'.[440] Nonetheless, Aristides was determined to follow the regimen Asclepius prescribed for him. However, even the extreme command of Asclepius that Aristides should draw blood from his forehead could not have been too unorthodox if a similar instruction was given to the Roman senator Sedatius, who, according to Aristides, complied willingly.[441] Moreover, Aristides' choice to site the case of Ischyron proves that he himself saw the therapeutic procedures of others as the appropriate context for his own experiences. It appears that the medical discourse in the temple was well-suited to the experiences of Aristides. Both the lack of a clear distinction between symptoms and a disease and the absence of a fully developed scientific paradigm meant there were not two mutually exclusive medical discourses—that of the temple and that of physicians. As eccentric as it seems to us, the behaviour of Aristides lay well within Graeco-Roman medical practices.

The temple of Asclepius provided Aristides with a medical discourse that was broad enough in its scope to include his religious experiences, alongside affiliated disciplines such as divination and dream-interpretation.[442] This does not merely mean that some of Aristides' physical symptoms and pathologies, such as choking, were understood to have been induced by a deity, but that Aristides' conceptualisation of being ill was an intrinsic aspect of a broader conceptual scheme of a religious nature, or so the reader is led to believe. Indeed, some of Aristides' healing experiences at the

---

439 References are collected and discussed by Nutton (2004); Jackson (1988); Penso (1984).

440 οἵ τε γὰρ νεωκόροι ἐν τούτῳ ὄντες ἡλικίας καὶ πάντες οἱ περὶ τὸν θεὸν θεραπευταὶ καὶ τάξεις ἔχοντες ὡμολόγουν ἀεὶ δή ποτε μηδένα πω τῶν πάντων συνειδέναι τοσαῦτα τμηθέντα, πλήν γε Ἰσχύρωνος, εἶναι δ' ἐν τοῖς παράδοξον τό γ' ἐκείνου, ἀλλὰ καὶ ὣς ὑπερβάλλειν τὸ καθ' ἡμᾶς ἄνευ τῶν ἄλλων παραδόξων. Aristid. *Or*. 48. 47 K.

441 Aristid. *Or*. 48. 48 K.

442 See the sections 'The Graeco-Roman health-care system' and 'The sick, medicine and physicians in the world of the *Sacred Tales*' above.

Asclepieion can only be defined as psychosomatic or spiritual. For example, in the years 145–146 CE, having been ordered by the god to resume his engagement in rhetoric and in particular lyric verse,[443] Aristides spent some time maintaining a chorus of boys and, as noted above, Aristides believed the singing of the boys cured his pains.[444] On another occasion Aristides tells a story of how he had a vision of Lysias, when he was sick with a 'very grave tertian fever' (ἔκαμνον γὰρ τριταίῳ οἵῳ βαπυτάτῳ).[445] On that day the attack was not followed by fever and Aristides says that 'at this time the disease was ended'.[446] Thus we find that the explanatory model Aristides used to comprehend the sudden improvement of his health did not exclude divine intervention and indeed included a particular understanding of the nature of dreams and dream-interpretation which provided Aristides with the kind of support contemporary scientific medicine could not. Furthermore, the therapeutic qualities of lyric verse and the appearance of Lysias linked Aristides to the glorious tradition of Greek orators and suggested that the god prescribed this quality of oratory to Aristides' medicine.[447] Likewise, these dreams marked Greek literature as the driving force of Aristides' aretalogical narrative of recuperation and, having a deity to induce it, it is also a narrative of redemption.

Throughout the winter of 145–146 CE Aristides' body was very weak and he could not leave his room for long periods of time.[448] In addition, there were various symptoms in relation to Aristides' teeth and ears, a general throbbing of his pulse, and an inability to hold food.[449] Aristides suffered from a fierce pain in his head and was unable to recline at night. In spite of all these hardships Aristides' faith did not weaken and in the spring of 146 CE he followed the god's command and journeyed to convalesce in Aliani.[450] While there his condition deteriorated with severe indigestion which led

---

[443] Aristid. *Or*. 50. 38 K.

[444] καὶ ὁπότε ἢ πνίγεσθαι συμβαίνοι, τοῦ τραχήλου ταθέντος ἐξαίφνης ἢ τοῦ στομάχου καταστάντος εἰς ἀπορίας, ἤ τις ἄλλη γένοιτο ἄπορος προσβολή, παρὼν ἂν Θεόδοτος ὁ ἰατρὸς καὶ μεμνημένος τῶν ἐνυπνίων ἐκέλευε τοὺς παῖδας ᾄδειν τῶν μελῶν, καὶ μεταξὺ ᾀδόντων λάθρα τις ἐγίγνετο ῥᾳστώνη, ἔστι δ' ὅτε καὶ παντελῶς ἀπῄει πᾶν τὸ λυποῦν. Aristid. *Or*. 50. 38 K.

[445] Aristid. *Or*. 50. 59 K.

[446] ἐπῄει δὲ ἡ τῆς καταβολῆς ἡμέρα καὶ ὁ πυρετὸς οὐκ ἐπεγένετο, ἀλλ' ἐλύθη τὸ νόσημα ἐν τούτῳ. Aristid. *Or*. 50. 59 K.

[447] Furthermore, the very name of Lysias also functioned as a cognate of the Greek λύσις i.e. release.

[448] Aristid. *Or*. 48. 34, 51, 56 K.

[449] Aristid. *Or*. 48. 57 K.

[450] Aristid. *Or*. 49. 1 K.

to breathing difficulties.[451] However, on the way back to Smyrna Aristides' condition improved and the god sent him a dream proclaiming that he was cured.[452]

Back in Pergamum in September 147 CE, after a long fever in the winter of 146/7 CE, the physician Satyrus, whom Aristides entitled 'a sophist of no mean rank', visited Aristides.[453] Having learned that Asclepius prescribed Aristides many purges (κάθαρσις) of blood, the physician ordered him to stop and not to undermine his body. Instead Satyrus prescribed an ointment for Aristides to put on his stomach and abdomen. As noted earlier, Aristides did not give preference to the authority of the famous physician and kept on purging blood, but he did use the ointment. Thus one can definitely see a hierarchy here—Aristides only followed remedies and regimen prescribed by physicians which were not in opposition to those of Asclepius—but it was a hierarchy which did not *a priori* exclude all secondary options. Later in October 147 CE, when Aristides was taken to the warm springs of Lebenus he used Satyrus' ointment, but only after explicitly stating that he saw no contradiction between the physician's prescription and that of Asclepius.[454] The application of the ointment did not agree with Aristides. He reported an unpleasant cold feeling.[455] Nevertheless Aristides persevered only to develop 'a terrible chest cold' (καὶ οὕτω δὴ τό τε στῆθος ψύχεται ψύξιν).[456] The god explained that it was consumption (καὶ ὁ θεὸς σημαίνει φθόην εἶναι).[457] On the following day he suffered what appears to be a migraine and his jaws were locked together.[458]

Aristides was often forced to choose between the treatment options of Asclepius and those of a physician. As has been said before, it was not uncommon for a physician to have to earn his patient's confidence, either in competition with other physicians or with temple-medicine,[459] but it seems that winning Aristides' trust had very little to do with scientific or methodological questions. The *Sacred Tales* do not record any evidence of such debates between Asclepius and the physicians. Moreover, the vocabulary

---

451 Aristid. *Or.* 49. 1 K.
452 Aristid. *Or.* 49. 5 K.
453 καὶ ἦν δὴ ὁ ἰατρὸς Σάτυρος ἐν Περγάμῳ κατὰ τοῦτον τὸν χρόνον σοφιστής, ὡς ἐλέγετο, οὐ τῶν ἀγεννῶν. Aristid. *Or.* 49. 8 K.
454 Aristid. *Or.* 49. 10–12 K.
455 Aristid. *Or.* 49. 11 K.
456 Aristid. *Or.* 49. 11 K.
457 'And the god showed it is to be consumption'. Aristid. *Or.* 49. 11 K.
458 Aristid. *Or.* 49. 11 K.
459 Cf. Gal. 17.137.7–12 K.

and the semantic network with which Aristides perceived and described his pathologies and treatments indicate that he felt religion and medicine were closely related. For instance in his account of the winter of 148/9 CE Aristides described suffering from a tumour of extraordinary size. Aristides' groin was distended, everything was swollen and terrible pains ensued for some days. Aristides consulted a number of physicians and received many suggested courses of treatment including surgery and cauterisation by drug. Aristides decided not to accept any of the medical advice he was given, but to continue with the regimen Asclepius prescribed, which was 'to endure and foster the growth' (ἀντέχειν καὶ τρέφειν τὸν ὄγκον). Although the growth continued to increase, and in spite of much criticism from friends and physicians, Aristides still would not undergo surgery or cauterising drugs.[460] Instead Aristides followed the god's advice to hold firm and bear the present circumstances. This state of affairs lasted for four months during which time Aristides' head and upper intestinal tract were 'as comfortable as one could pray for' (ἐν δὲ τούτοις κεφαλὴ μὲν οὕτω κούφη καὶ τὰ ἄνω τῆς κοιλίας, ὡς ἂν μάλιστά τις εὔξαιτο).[461]

The regimen Asclepius prescribed to Aristides at this time included running unshod in wintertime, horseback riding, eating honey and acorns, and vomiting, all of which were common prescriptions of Asclepius.[462] Aristides had to fulfil these instructions while the growth was still of its full size and was spreading up to Aristides' navel. Only then did Asclepius prescribe a certain salt-containing drug, the particular nature of which Aristides does not remember, and when this drug was applied the growth quickly disappeared in one single night. This event changed the relationship Aristides had with his physicians. The doctors stopped their criticism, expressed extraordinary admiration of the god, and said 'it was some other greater disease, which he secretly cured' (καὶ ὡς ἕτερόν τι ἄρα ἦν μεῖζον, ὃ λάθρᾳ ἰᾶτο).[463]

The *Sacred Tales* are the only source we have for Aristides' malady, his disposition as a sick man, his attitude towards physicians and their attitude towards him. This therefore makes an evaluation of the reliability of his work as evidence for his own medical history, and the history of medicine

---

460 On the role of physicians and on the role of withholding detail of the drug used see Petsalis-Diomidis (2010) 113.

461 Aristid. *Or.* 47. 61–64 K.

462 Cf. M. Ant. 5.8.1: Ὁποῖόν τί ἐστι τὸ λεγόμενον, ὅτι· συνέταξεν ὁ Ἀσκληπιὸς τούτῳ ἱππασίαν ἢ ψυχρολουσίαν ἢ ἀνυποδησίαν, τοιοῦτόν ἐστι καὶ τό· συνέταξε τούτῳ ἡ τῶν ὅλων φύσις νόσον ἢ πήρωσιν ἢ ἀποβολὴν ἢ ἄλλο τι τῶν τοιούτων.

463 Aristid. *Or.* 47. 67 K.

in general, difficult to establish. His account is not without ambiguities. For example, Aristides reports that the healing of his growth persuaded his physicians to acknowledge the validity of Asclepius' treatment. However he goes on to say that these very same physicians thought that the loose skin where the growth used to be must be removed surgically. This description of such a miraculous healing process makes it difficult to accept Aristides' testimony at face-value and he himself indicates the doubts that still existed amongst the physicians as they continued to advocate a surgical solution. It is true that Aristides has them say that this advice did not contradict the god's regimen since 'now the god's part had been done' (πάντως δὲ ἤδη πεπρᾶχθαι τά γε τού θεοῦ),[464] but it is also possible that they did not share his zeal and conviction. In any case Aristides disagreed with the physicians and continued to follow Asclepius' regimen, which commanded him to smear an egg on the loose skin. He reported that this remedy finally cured him: 'After a few days had passed, no one was able to find on which thigh the tumour had been' (ὥστε ὀλίγων ἡμερῶν παρελθουσῶν οὐδεὶς οἷός τ' ἦν εὑρεῖν ἐν ὁποτέρῳ μηρῷ τὸ φῦμα ἐκεῖνο ἐγένετο).[465]

Aristides continued to consult both Asclepius and physicians. On most occurrences he approached both and then made a decision. In his report of around February 148 CE, while at his family estates, Aristides experienced an unbearable headache, a convulsion and a fever.[466] A doctor was summoned who concluded that Aristides should be fed. Aristides, however, decided not to yield to the doctor's prescription and instead to follow a command he received in a dream during the following night in which he was instructed to pay homage to the statue of Zeus there.[467] He followed this order and he was subsequently cured.[468]

Aristides' ailments did not end at this point. In late January 148 CE Aristides was still consumptive.[469] Asclepius himself diagnosed him and instructed Asclepiacus, the temple warden, to cure Aristides' consumption,

---

464 Ibid.

465 Aristid. *Or.* 47. 68 K.

466 Aristid. *Or.* 49. 16–17 K.

467 Aristides' choice to make a pilgrimage to a statue of Zeus, rather than Asclepius, in order to procure divine remedy is an interesting one. Though Aristides was definitely aware of the traditional picture of the Greek pantheon with Zeus as the father of the universe and the rest of the gods as deriving their forces from him, their creator and father (see below the chapter 'reconsidering private religions'), hence perceiving Asclepius to draw his powers from the mightier Zeus, Aristides, as he depicted himself in the *Sacred Tales*, was particularly devoted to Asclepius.

468 Aristid. *Or.* 49. 20 K.

469 Ibid.

catarrh, and stomach ailment.[470] A report from the following month (February 148 CE) exemplifies how limited Aristides' understanding of human anatomy was, and how indiscriminate he was in using both metaphors and literal descriptions relating to his condition. In the *Tales* Aristides gives an account of a dream that Neritus, one of his foster-fathers, had about him. The dream can be dated to February 148 CE. In the dream Asclepius and Telesphorus tell Neritus that it was necessary to replace all Aristides' bones and nerves, 'for the existing ones had failed' (τὰ γὰρ ὄντα ἀπειρηκέναι).[471] Such an extreme procedure was not, of course, undertaken. Asclepius explained that there was no need to remove the bones and nerves, but rather that a certain change was needed in the existing bones and nerves.[472] The cure the god gave to achieve this correction was unsalted olive oil three times a day. Aristides does not tell us if the olive oil was to be consumed or smeared. The answer might have been written in Aristides' extensive notes to which he referred his keener readership elsewhere.[473] Regardless of the nature of the application, Aristides followed the god's regimen and it proved helpful.[474] From this episode it appears that Aristides was not fully familiar with the actual function of the skeleton or the nervous system of the human body, and that he did not expect the god's regimen to be based on any logical or medical connection between pathology and its cure. This observation should be used to make a wider claim regarding the Graeco-Roman health care system. It appears that the grid of knowledge which defined the realm of the medical discourse in Aristides' day did not force a dichotomy between literal and metaphorical anatomical descriptions, which, in turn, meant patients were not required to have mechanical explanations to their ailments, of the type which are provable by experiment. Using Kuhn's terminology, it meant the absence of a medical paradigm.

Aristides viewed the relationship between himself and the healing deity of Asclepius more in the terms of a physician and his patient than that of a worshipper and his god. For Aristides, Asclepius was both a god and his physician. According to the *Sacred Tales*, this attitude did not force Aristides to renounce all services of other physicians. On the contrary, the picture that emerges from the *Sacred Tales* is a world in which temple

470 Aristid. *Or*. 49. 14 K.
471 Aristid. *Or*. 49. 15 K.
472 Ibid.
473 Aristides explicitly encouraged his readers to consult these notes: Aristid. *Or*. 48.1–3 K.
474 Aristid. *Or*. 49. 15 K.

medicine and scientific medicine complement each other, share a common professional language and acknowledge both the validity of each other and their therapeutic measures.

Wider Contexts

By setting the medical history of Aelius Aristides within a wider context it is possible to determine whether his history, as recorded in his *Sacred Tales*, reflected habits which were typical of his age or whether it is the history of an eccentric individual. In order to provide such a contextualisation it is necessary to address two issues. The first is the question of how common was Aristides' approach towards Asclepius and his cult, the role of dreams in his medical treatment and his chosen treatment options. The second is to locate Aristides' health and his comprehension of it in relation to the understandings of health and sickness which dominated the world he inhabited.

The religious means that Aristides chose as the most appropriate to fight his illness, and the particular influence Asclepius had upon him, were far from being eccentric. The cult of Asclepius was widespread as the archaeological evidence from the various Asclepieiea and the plethora of dedications clearly show.[475] Strabo, for example, writes of Epidaurus that 'this city is not without distinction, and particularly because of the epiphany of Asclepius, who is believed to cure diseases of every kind and always has his temple full of the sick, and also of the votive tablets on which the treatments are recorded, just as at Cos, and Tricca'.[476] Moreover, the patients in the Pergamene Asclepieion were usually keen to follow the god's instructions,[477] unlike their more reserved disposition towards physicians, which was a cause of concern for Galen.[478]

---

[475] Cf. Jost (1985); Sherwin-White (1978) 334–339; Graf (1992); Roesch (1985); Aleshire (1989); Tomilson (1983); Roebuck (1953); Lang (1977); Rubensohn (1902) 199–238; Roesch (1982) 171–179.

[476] καὶ αὕτη δ' οὐκ ἄσημος ἡ πόλις καὶ μάλιστα διὰ τὴν ἐπιφάνειαν τοῦ Ἀσκληπιοῦ θεραπεύειν νόσους παντοδαπὰς πεπιστευμένου, καὶ τὸ ἱερὸν πλῆρες ἔχοντος ἀεὶ τῶν τε καμνόντων καὶ τῶν ἀνακειμένων πινάκων, ἐν οἷς ἀναγεγραμμέναι τυγχάνουσιν αἱ θεραπεῖαι, καθάπερ ἐν Κῷ τε καὶ Τρίκκῃ. Str. 8.6.15.

[477] Cf. Müller (1987) 194.

[478] οὕτω γέ τοι καὶ παρ' ἡμῖν ἐν Περγάμῳ τοὺς θεραπευομένους ὑπὸ τοῦ θεοῦ πειθομένους ὁρῶμεν αὐτῷ πεντεκαίδεκα πολλάκις ἡμέραις προστάξαντι μηδ' ὅλως πιεῖν, οἳ τῶν ἰατρῶν μηδενὶ προστάττοντι πείθονται. μεγάλην γὰρ ἔχει ῥοπὴν εἰς τὸ πάντα ποιῆσαι τὰ προστταττόμενα τὸ πεπεῖσθαι τὸν κάμνοντα βεβαίως ἀκολουθήσειν ὠφέλειαν ἀξιόλογον αὐτῷ. 'In this way also among

The popularity of both the cult of Asclepius and of temple-medicine in the Graeco-Roman world during the high empire is demonstrated by the attendance at the Asclepieia of high-ranking Romans and Greeks alike.[479] It is reported that all of Asia flocked to the temple of Asclepius of Pergamum,[480] where a temple of Asclepius had existed since the fourth century BCE.[481] The popularity of the Pergamene Asclepieion is obvious from the extensive epigraphical evidence found in the temple.[482] By the second century CE the cult of Asclepius was widespread throughout Graeco-Roman society, not least among the educated. By the time Aristides was writing and worshipping, the Asclepieion was the most popular place of worship in Pergamum,[483] and Martial used *Pergamus deus* as a synonym for Asclepius.[484] Moreover, the inclination of Roman emperors to bestow benefactions on the Greek cities resulted in some of the era's most beautiful buildings, including some which were temples of Asclepius.[485]

The new second-century temple of Pergamum was built during the latter years of Hadrian and the early years of Antoninus Pius by L. Cuspius Pactumeius Rufinus (cos. ord. 142 CE),[486] who was a friend of Aristides (*Or.* 50. 28, 43, 83, 84, 107 K) and of Galen's first teacher Satyrus, in turn an acquaintance of Aristides who consulted him on medical issues.[487] The grand scale of the works suggests an imperial guiding hand.[488] Other noteworthy benefactors of the Pergamene Asclepieion were Aulus Claudius Charax,[489] and Aris-

---

us in Pergamum we see that those who are taken care of by the god obey him when he often orders them not to drink anything at all for fifteen days; people who do not obey any of the physicians. For the fact that the ill person hopes that some kind of considerable help will certainly accompany him, this has great strength in order to make him [i.e. the sick] perform all that has been prescribed'.' Gal. 17.137.7–12 K.

479 See above, p. 87.

480 Cf. Philostr. *VA* 4.34; Aristid. *Or.* 23. 16 K.

481 Str. 2.26.8; Philostr. *VA* 4. 34. Edelstein and Edelstein vol. ii. (1945) 249.

482 Habicht (1969) is essential. See also Hoffmann (1998) 47.

483 Habicht (1969) 6–18; Hoffmann (1998) 41.

484 Mart. 9.16.2.

485 The renaissance of the Pergamene Asclepieion is documented by inscriptions (which list the privileges bestowed on its priests and are indicative of imperial favour).

486 Habicht (1969) 3.9–11.

487 The remodelling of the Asclepieion probably took place between Hadrian's two visits to the Roman province of Asia. For dating see Habicht (1969) 6–18. Aristid. *Or.* 49. 8–11 K. Swain (1996) 257. Rufinus: Halfman (1979) no. 66; Habicht (1969) 23 ff., no. 2; *PIR*[2] C 1637. Satyrus and Rufinus: Gal. 2.224.17–225 K; Bowersock (1969) 60–61. Date of reconstruction of the temple of Asclepius: Habicht (1969) 10–11; Le Glay (1976) 347–372. On the actual new temple itself see Petsalis-Diomidis (2010) 194–202.

488 *I. Perg.* XI,3, 30–76; *I. Perg.* VIII,3, 11–14; Hoffmann (1998) 46–47.

489 L. Cuspius Pactumeius Rufinus dedicated the temple of Zeus Asclepius: Behr (1968) 27–28; Aristid. *Or.* 47. 31 K; Magie (1950) 1494; Habicht (1969) 9–10, 142. A. Claudius Charax

tides' friend, the consular Vitrasius Pollio.[490] The remodelled Asclepieion was dedicated to the universal god Zeus-Asclepius and was, as Habicht argues, designed to form a counterpart to the old and local traditions. Aristides himself distinguished between the old Hellenistic temple and that of Rufinus.[491] Likewise, the architecture chosen for the new annexes of the temple was a declaration of deliberate contrast to its Hellenistic counterpart. The Zeus-Asclepius temple is a miniature replica of the Pantheon in Rome, which suggests that it was intended to serve a similar function or to instigate similar reactions.[492] With its large domed roof it must have appealed to every visitor, particularly its Roman convalescents, as an embodiment of the very latest Roman architecture.[493] The fact that the Zeus-Asclepius temple was such a celebrated and distinguished building is indicative of the central role played by the cult of Asclepius in Graeco-Roman society at this time. Aristides' decision to consult Asclepius therefore cannot simply be termed the actions of an eccentric, and must be seen in the context of his cultural and social milieu.

Perhaps the most striking feature of Aristides' medical history is the seminal role he allowed dreams to play within it. All through his search for cure, from physicians, through the temple warden Asclepiacus, to Asclepius himself, dreams never ceased to guide Aristides' choices of treatment options. It appears from the *Sacred Tales* that dreams often functioned as the medium through which the god communicated medical prescriptions to Aristides. In August 148 CE, to name but one incident, Aristides had a cryptic dream, which included a royal ointment.[494] As detailed above, Aristides consulted Asclepiacus, the temple warden, who interpreted the dream, the ointment was found and the cleansing (κάθαρσις) was completed. However,

from Pergamum and a contemporary of Aristides who was a priest and a consul in 147 CE. In addition to his beneficiary activities in Pergamum, Charax also composed a universal history in forty books, covering especially Greek and, from book twelve, Roman history up to the period of 'Nero and his successors' (*Suda* s.v.). The work was later summarised and used by Stephanus of Byzantium under the title *Chroniká*. The fragments relate mostly to mythological times, as it was mainly his euhemeristic and allegorical interpretation of the myths that the Byzantines drew on C. *FGrH* 103 (comm. and add. to 2 AB in 3 B, 741f.). K. Meister in: *DNP* 3, 191. On Charax see Andrei (1984).

490 Habicht (1969) 3.10, 103–106.

491 Cf. Aristid. Or. 42.4; 47.45; 50.46 K; Jones (1998) 69.

492 Petsalis-Diomidis (2010) 194.

493 Hoffmann (1998) 49.

494 Aristid. *Or.* 49. 21 K.

as noted earlier in this chapter, Aristides' approach to dreams was far from being innovative or unusual. The interest of ancient medicine in dreams in general, and an understanding of dreams as functioning as signs or symptoms that should initiate a medical response in particular, lay at the heart of Graeco-Roman medical thought with precedents that went back to the Hippocratic corpus.[495]

Although Aristides left no treatise in which he discusses the nature of dreams, his many dream-reports imply that he shared the view that the gods can indeed send dreams and that if the gods send a dream containing medical advice it is to be taken literally.[496] For instance, on 20 January 166 CE Aristides dreamt that 'after my food was not digested properly, I consulted Zosimus, my foster-father, about bathing and asked him if it were necessary to bathe more. But he did not agree. After this I bathed and then had stomach trouble, and said to Zosimus, "was it necessary to fast?" and he said, "it was necessary"'.[497] Aristides followed the dream's command and fasted. On the next day (January 21) Aristides vomited again in the evening and then he dreamt 'that a bone was annoying me and there was a need to expel it, and a notion of drawing blood from the ankles'. Aristides did so and he records that 'there was a very light discharge'.[498] Aristides did not look for clinical sense in the god's commands even when they included extreme measures, probably because his perception of human physiology was inadequate and because his understanding of medical care as a whole was not this way inclined. Even more importantly, it is nowhere suggested that Aristides' environment encouraged him to look for a clinical explanation to his condition.

Another opportunity to contextualise Aristides' medical history in general and his choices of treatment options in particular is provided through examining his approach to his diet. A reader of the *Sacred Tales* cannot fail to notice the seminal role played by food and diet in Aristides' medical history. On the advice of gods and men he refrained from eating certain things, induced vomiting and often fasted, all for medical purposes. His behaviour

---

495 See section 'Aristides, dreams and Graeco-Roman medicine'.

496 A statement explicitly made by Artemidorus, Artem. iv. 22. p, 255 l. 9.

497 ἐδόκουν ἐφθαρμένης μοι τῆς τροφῆς συμβουλεύεσθαι περὶ λουτροῦ Ζωσίμῳ τῷ τροφεῖ καὶ ἐρωτᾶν εἰ δέοι πλείω λούσασθαι. τὸν δὲ οὐ συμφῆσαι. μετὰ δὲ τοῦτο λελοῦσθαί γε καὶ τῆς γαστρὸς φαύλως ἔχειν, καὶ φάναι πρὸς τὸν Ζώσιμον, ἔδει γὰρ ἠσιτηκέναι; καὶ τὸν εἰπεῖν, ἔδει. Aristid. *Or.* 47. 27 K.

498 καὶ τῆς ἐπιούσης ἤμουν πάλιν εἰς ἑσπέραν. ἦν δὲ τὸ ὄναρ ὡς ὀστοῦ γε ἐγκειμένου καὶ δέον ἐκβαλεῖν, ἔννοια δὲ καὶ αἵματος ἀφαιρέσεως ἀπὸ τῶν σφυρῶν. Aristid. *Or.* 47. 28 K.

was, however, not at all uncommon. Diet was a central element in Graeco-Roman medicine. Writing at the time of the emperor Claudius, Scribonianus Largus summed up the steps of medical care: first came diet, then drugs, and finally either cautery or surgery.[499] Plutarch thought that a good physician was someone who used sleep and diet rather than violent drugs to affect cures.[500] Ancient medicine saw diet as vital for health since food could cause disease or restore health through its effects on the balance of the humours.[501] Galen himself composed a treatise *On the Powers of Foods*. In this treatise foods are carefully classified according to their powers. Aristides' dietary habits were in tune with this line of thought.

Aristides took great care to conform to Asclepius' commands in his dietary habits. In 170/1 CE he reports that he abstained from eating 'all living things, and all greens, except wild ones and lettuce, and I have abstained from all sweet meats. Now occasionally he has commanded me to eat a whole chicken, and I have done so ... for six years I have abstained from all fish. I do not know how long from pork ... he [i.e. Asclepius] has kept me completely from fish sauce'.[502] Aristides followed a god-ordered regimen of strict diet from the very the earliest time Asclepius approached him. Already in the spring of 149 CE the god prohibited him in a dream from eating beef.[503]

Aristides' dietary habits, of which the better part were induced by a deity, call to mind other religious dietary interdictions and precepts, which existed in the Graeco-Roman world,[504] but were seen as common criteria of ethnicity rather than aspects of medical discourse.[505] Particularly noteworthy here is the Jewish example where religious dietary regulations were perceived by those practising Judaism to be associated with health-care,[506] but by others, such as Tacitus, as a symptom of anti-social behaviour.[507] Hence,

---

499 Scrib. Larg. Intr. 6. For the background of this rather forgotten author see Baldwin (1992) and Hamilton (1986).

500 Plut. *Mor.* 73d.

501 Grant (2000) 7.

502 ἦν δέ τις χρόνος οὗτος, ὅτ' ἐμψύχων τε ἀπειχόμην, πλὴν ἀλεκτρυόνος, καὶ λαχάνων ἁπάντων, πλὴν ἀγρίων καὶ θριδακίνης, καὶ τραγημάτων δ' ἀπειχόμην πάντων ... ἰχθύων δὲ καὶ ἓξ ἔτη πάντων ἀπεσχόμην· ὑείων δὲ οὐκ οἶδα ὁπόσον τι ... καὶ μὴν γάρου γε εἶρξε καθάπαξ. Aristid. *Or.* 49. 34–35 K.

503 Aristid. *Or.* 48. 37 K.

504 Isaac (2004) 450–492; Schäfer (1997) 81–86.

505 Hdt. 3.1, 23; 9.82.

506 All dietary regulations were collected in the sections in the Talmud that discussed dietary regulations—דיני כשרות. There is no need, however, to discuss them here in detail. They were inaccessible to those who could not read Hebrew or Aramaic.

507 Tac. *Hist.* 5.5.1.

dietary and cleansing habits were meaningful, important, and crucial in various ways in the Graeco-Roman world. The fact that Aristides saw no need for explanations is in itself a strong argument for the familiarity of the ruling class of the Graeco-Roman world with these habits, that they viewed them in a medical context, and for the ability of the *Sacred Tales* to represent common behaviour in Aristides' Graeco-Roman circles.

Finally, the general health of the Roman world, both in itself and as seen by contemporaries, is an inherent part of the context of Aristides' medical history. Indeed, the *Sacred Tales*' account of the second half of the 160s reveals another significant point, namely how Aristides' health was also affected by the health of the empire as a whole. The return of Lucius Verus and the Roman legions from the eastern frontier in the mid-160s brought the plague into Rome, and it remained endemic for many years to come.[508] The biographer of Lucius says that 'it was his fate to bring the plague with him to those provinces through which he made his return journey, right up to Rome'.[509] Galen, who was in Rome in 166 CE, fled the city in fear of the plague and returned to Pergamum.[510] Religious explanations were common and added to an overall air of anxiety: for example, the plague was a result of opening a golden casket containing the dread vapour in the temple of Apollo at Seleucia.[511] Avidius Cassius, the Roman general and future usurper who wrongfully sacked Seleucia was also to blame for breaking a treaty. Lucian has the false prophet Alexander selling magic charms, exploiting the general anxiety.[512] Ammianus Marcellinus and Orosius attest that the horrific sights were not forgotten centuries later.[513] Aristides was, of course, aware of the plague in the summer of 165 CE.[514] After many of his household were struck by it, Aristides himself was infected. He describes it as 'terrible burning of a bilious mixture, which troubled me continuously day and night, and I was prevented from taking nourishment and my strength failed'.[515]

---

508 For the devastating impact of the Antonine plague see Duncan-Jones (1996). Galen himself escaped Rome because of the plague (see above, p. 66). For the impact of the plague on Aristides and his household see above, pp. 88–89.

509 *Fuit eius fati ut in eas provincias per quas rediit Romam usque luem secum deferre videretur*. SHA, *Verus*, 8.1.

510 R.J. and M.L. Littman (1973) 243–255, discuss the evidence of Galen.

511 SHA, *Verus*, 8.1–2.

512 Lucian, *Alex*. 36. For an analysis of Lucian rhetoric here see Petsalis-Diomidis (2010) 42–59.

513 Amm. Marc. 31.6.24; Oros. 7.15.5–6; 7.27.7.

514 Aristid. *Or*. 48. 37–38 K.

515 καὶ κατελήφθην ὑπὸ δεινοῦ πυρὸς χολῆς παντοίας, ἣ συνεχῶς νύκτα καὶ ἡμέραν ἠνώχλει, καὶ τῆς τροφῆς ἀπεκεκλείμην καὶ ἡ δύναμις κατελέλυτο. Aristid. *Or*. 48. 39 K.

He was then instructed by Asclepius and by Athena to take an enema of Attic honey, and there was a purge of the bile. After this came curatives and nourishment and finally Aristides recovered.[516]

Placing the medical history of Aelius Aristides, as portrayed in the *Sacred Tales*, in the context of the social, cultural and political climate in which he lived demonstrates that rather than trying to find an eccentric or alternative remedy Aristides conceived of his illness and sought medical help in the places his world designated as most suitable for these purposes. Aristides' choices of treatment options from those available to him suggest an erudite and careful approach rather than one which was superstitious and sporadic. The physicians he consulted included some of the most distinguished health-care providers in the Graeco-Roman world and the cult of Asclepius was also a natural choice for a Greek in the province of Asia during the high empire. Aristides' dietary habits, his identification of those capable of helping him (men and gods alike), as well as his understanding of the dream-mechanism and its utility in medical care reflect many of the most common modes of thought of his age. Furthermore, the health of the Empire at this time was also responsible for some sense of anxiety in the *Sacred Tales*. The great plague of 165 CE left a devastating trail of death in Asia Minor, which did not exclude Aristides' household. The plague was but one contributory factor to a general mood of disquiet and a widely held interest in bodily grievances and disease.[517] The medical history of Aristides, much like the *Sacred Tales* themselves, should be seen as a product of its time. They should be read as a layman's testimony of the health care system which prevailed in his day. His descriptions should be used to map the power structure in the field of health care. His narrative of the treatments he underwent and his coming to terms with his condition are indicative of the pre-paradigmatic state of medicine in his day, not of the personal experiences of an individual.

A study of the *Sacred Tales*, which leads towards a medical history of Aristides, must take into account the fact that this work was intended to be read and that it was, indeed, published. Its ancient readers, such as Philostratus and Libanius, Sopater and Synesius did not find it eccentric or untrustworthy.[518] On the contrary, they noted Aristides' *Sacred Tales* as an exemplary

---

516 Aristid. *Or*. 48. 42–44 K.

517 It is noteworthy that Aristides decided to write the *Sacred Tales* only after the plague.

518 I discussed the composition of the *Sacred Tales*, their purpose and impact on their ancient readers above.

record of one's medical history and of proper writing.[519] It is therefore safe to assume that as far as a history of medicine is concerned, the *Sacred Tales* were representative enough of their contemporary medical discourse even if they appear dissimilar to works of physicians.[520] Bearing in mind that the *Sacred Tales* were written by a patient, not by a doctor, and that Aristides was not trying to write a medical treatise, historians of medicine should nonetheless value the *Sacred Tales* as an exceptional document of a sick person's experience of seeking medical help and being treated.[521]

Perhaps the most striking feature of Aristides' depiction of his ailments, his dreams, and the process of healing is that he perceived his disease as essentially a collection of symptoms rather than as the result of a certain ailment. For instance he did not report suffering from a new disease after being struck by the plague. On the contrary, there is a sense of continuity in his account, even if the symptoms do mark a clinical shift in his condition. In addition, Aristides' chronology of his illness, which begins at 142 CE and continues to document his years of sickness, does so without referring to any fundamental shift in his medical condition.[522] In fact, Aristides never makes any attempt to grasp the nature of his disease and he does not discuss his condition in general medical or scientific terms. On January 6, 166 CE Aristides dreams 'that some Parthians had got me in their power, and one of them approached me and made as if to brand me. Next he inserted a finger in my throat and poured in something, according to some native custom, and named it "sour-food". Later I recounted these things as they had appeared in the dream. And the audience marvelled and said that the cause of my thirst and inability to drink was this, that my food turned sour. Because of this vomiting was indicated and the Parthian ordered that I abstain from bathing today and produce one servant as a witness of this'.[523]

---

519 See above, chap. 1, sec. 3, 'The ancient readers of the *Sacred Tales*'.

520 For the existence of a medical discourse above, chap. 2, sec. 2. 'The sick, medicine, and physicians in the *Sacred Tales*'.

521 As agrgued convisingly by Horstmanshoff (1990), (2004).

522 E.g. c. December 22, 152 CE Aristides counts ten years of being sick. Aristid. *Or.* 50. 1; 52.1 K.

523 τινας τῶν βαρβάρων ἐγκρατεῖς γεγενῆσθαί μου, καί τινα αὐτῶν ἐπιέναι μοι
καὶ δόξαν παρασχεῖν ὡς στίξοντα· ἔπειτα καθεῖναι τὸν δάκτυλον οὑτωσὶ μέχρι τοῦ λαιμοῦ, καί τι ἐγχέαι, κατὰ δή τινα ἐπιχώριον νόμον, ὀνομάσαι δὲ αὐτὸ ὀξυσιτίαν· ταῦτα δὲ ὕστερον ὡς ὄναρ διηγεῖσθαι καὶ τοὺς ἀκούοντας θαυμάζειν καὶ λέγειν ὡς ἄρα τοῦτο αἴτιον εἴη τοῦ διψῆν μὲν, μὴ δύνασθαι δὲ πιεῖν, τὸ τρέπεσθαι εἰς ὄξος τὰ σιτία. ἐκ δὴ τούτου ἔμετός τε ἐδείκνυτο καὶ προσέταξεν ὁ βάρβαρος λουτροῦ τε ἀποσχέσθαι καὶ διάκονον ἕνα παραστήσασθαι. τὸ τήμερον εἶναι. Aristid. *Or.* 47. 9 K.

All that Aristides tells us after having this dream is that he refrained from bathing, vomiting and comfort, but there is nothing to suggest that this, or for that matter any other of his dreams, helped him to formulate a firmer notion of the nature of his physical condition, or that he saw all his symptoms as having a unified clinical meaning. This absence of an appreciation of cause-and-effect between symptoms and disease or between cure and disease, at least in a scientific sense, is further revealed in the way Aristides reports and interprets his dream of January 12, in which a bull pressed against his right knee. After waking up a small sore, like a carbuncle, had appeared there. Aristides felt that it seemed to be good for the upper part of the digestive tract.[524] However, he made no explanation of, or even inquiry into the connection between the bull, the knee, the sore and his digestion.[525]

Aristides took no particular interest in describing the physical manifestations of his illness *per se*. The reader is often left with the regimen the god prescribed without knowing what the medical condition was to begin with. This is the case in a comment from January 15 which discloses that Aristides was vomiting again in the evening according to a dream.[526] A few days later, on January 18, Aristides had a dream that 'someone said "Koiphi with wine". I immediately took it as medicine and considered whether it was necessary to apply it on my face or internally. And then when someone said that it would burn wherever it was applied, I thought it would be all the pre-eminently suitable to be a drug for cold. And somehow after this, I said to the priest that it was clear from what I had been reading that there would be no need to eat. Thereupon I intended to pass the day in fasting'. Having woken up, Aristides tells us, he spent the day fasting.[527] Aristides gives no indication of the symptoms he felt this treatment was supposed to cure.

Aristides' decision not to discuss his malady in general terms or to provide a medical explanation of either his condition or of the treatment he underwent could have resulted from literary considerations. As said before, the *Sacred Tales* were not written as a medical work.[528] It is a diary-like

524 Aristid. *Or.* 47. 14 K.

525 See above, p. 113.

526 Aristid. *Or.* 47. 21 K.

527 κἀκ τούτου δὴ ἐδόκουν εἰπεῖν τινὰ κοιφὶ μετὰ οἴνου· λαβεῖν τε δὴ εὐθὺς αὐτὸ ὡς ἴαμα καὶ σκοπεῖν εἴτε τῷ προσώπῳ δέοι προσθέσθαι εἴτε καὶ τοῖς ἐντός. καί τινος εἰπόντος ὅτι ἐπικάοι ὅπου ἐπιτεθείη, ἐνθυμηθῆναι ὡς ἐπιτηδείως ἔχοι παντὸς μᾶλλον ψύξεως εἶναι φάρμακον. καί πως ἐκ τούτων εἰπεῖν πρὸς τὸν ἱερέα ὅτι δῆλον ἦν ἐξ ὧν ἀνεγίγνωσκον ὅτι οὐχὶ δεήσοι φαγεῖν. καὶ δῆτα εὐθὺς εἶχον ἐν νῷ ὡς διατελέσων ἄσιτος τὴν ἡμέραν. Aristid. *Or.* 47. 26 K.

528 However, as shown by Roy Porter (1985) patients' dieries ate of profound importance to historians of medicine.

treatise commemorating the achievements of the saviour,[529] and a record of the providence of the god and the revelations of Asclepius to Aristides, which occurred after Aristides decided to submit himself to the god 'as to a doctor'.[530] However, a more plausible explanation of the paucity of medical explanations is that Aristides did not understand the mechanism of disease or medicine in this way. There is no consistent reference to cause and effect in his descriptions of symptoms and illness and no clinical logic (not just to a modern viewer, but that which one finds in ancient medical works as well) in the prescribed cures. The simplest explanation for this absence is that it was not part of Aristides' own explanatory model. Furthermore, a medical history of Aristides, as portrayed in the *Sacred Tales*, reveals no clear distinction between physicians and those who practiced temple medicine, either in the therapeutic measures they prescribed or in the professional language they used. Equally interesting, a taxonomy of magic versus science is nowhere to be found in the *Sacred Tales*. Science, as an explanatory model which focuses on a mechanistic explanation, must have been alien to Aristides' frame of thought.

Aristides' medical history discloses a distinctive aretalogical narrative of redemption. From Aristides' initial failure to find cure and recuperate without the god, through the inevitable recognition of the need for the divine in order for him to regain his health, the *Sacred Tales* depict an odyssey of a believer towards his faith. In this respect the role of Aristides' vocation is particularly interesting here, because his career follows a very similar path to his medical history. From an initial failure, which culminated in Aristides' first journey to Rome in 144 CE, through a period of training in the Pergamene Asclepieion and under Asclepius' supervision, tellingly entitled *cathedra*, towards a final success and glory, rhetoric was both Aristides' cure as much as it was his divine calling. Indeed it could be argued that Aristides' medical history, as portrayed in the *Sacred Tales*, is an orator's sophisticated attempt to glorify himself. Nonetheless, this medical history is historically valuable both for a history of Aristides himself and for a social history of Aristides' world.

529 Aristid. *Or.* 47. 1 K.
530 Aristid. *Or.* 47. 4 K.

Conclusion

In this chapter I have looked into society, disease and medicine in Aristides' *Sacred Tales*. More specifically, I have examined how the notion of illness is portrayed in the *Sacred Tales*, and how they conceived of medical intervention. In order to answer these questions I have enquired how these notions translated into actions, namely (i) what was the place society allocated to its sick; (ii) whom did the world of the *Sacred Tales* designate as authoritative in offering health-care and how was this authority accounted for; and finally (iii) what were the key characteristics of medical praxis. Having set the context by undertaking a broader look at medicine and dream-interpretation in classical antiquity, as well as explaining and applying sociological and anthropological concepts such as health-care systems and medical discourse, I have endeavoured to write a history of Aristides' malady. I was particularly interested in how Aristides' came to terms with his physiological symptoms; his special relationship with Asclepius; and his appeals to other health-care providers. In sum, I have asked to what extent the medical history of Aelius Aristides can be seen as representative of the health-care system of his day.

It is evident from the *Sacred Tales* themselves, as well as from a study of ancient medicine and the disciplines related to it, that the health-care system in Aristides' day was still anchored in other institutions and belief-systems, mainly philosophy, cosmology and religion. Galen himself argued that the finest doctors are also philosophers. According to Galen, the best physician 'possesses all the parts of philosophy: logic, natural science, and ethics'.[531] In fact, Galen demanded that physicians should engage in a study of philosophy as a fundamental part of their training.[532] Moreover, Galen did not present this demand as innovative. On the contrary, he imagined one tradition of philosophy and medicine which began with Hippocrates and passed through Plato, Aristotle and Chrysippus to Galen himself.[533] This was all part of Galen's perception of himself as a continuer of ancient orthodoxy.[534] It was the same Galen who acknowledged the importance of dreams in medical praxis and provides strong evidence for the popularity of the cult of Asclepius in the second century CE.[535]

531 Gal. *Opt. Med.* 1.60–61 K.
532 Gal. *Opt. Med.*
533 Barnes (1991) 51.
534 Galen, *Opt. Med.* 10. 309, 346; Barnes (1991) 52.
535 Dreams in medical practice: Gal. 16.222 K; the popularity of the Pergamene Asclepieion:

said before, Galen was the first amongst ancient medical authors to think of symptoms, diseases and affection in terms of one hermetic system, subjected to a rigid causal structure. None of his predecessors endeavoured to either draw a distinction between health and disease or between disease, symptoms and affection. Furthermore, no attempt had been made by any of Galen's predecessors to systematically classify *all* symptoms and associate them with *each* disease. When Galen faced this task in his works *De morborum differentiis*,[543] *De causis morborum*,[544] *De symptomatum differentiis*,[545] *De symptomatum causis*,[546] it was a ground-breaking enterprise whose aftermath is still present today. However, in Aristides' day such views were far removed from medical practice and medical discourse, all the more so from the point of view of the patient who was unlikely to envisage his illness as an intellectual odyssey. On the contrary, Aristides looked for practical solutions and he turned to those whom tradition sanctioned as most able—physicians, gymnastic trainers and priests. Only hindsight makes Aristides' comprehension of his illness and its narration extreme. To a contemporary, Aristides' choices and thoughts must have seemed far more reasonable.

Aristides' experiences of being ill and seeking medical help reveal much of his own disposition, but they also illuminate some of the main features of the Graeco-Roman health-care system, which shaped his experiences into their particular form. As has been noted above, the formulation of illness as a psychological experience cannot be other than a cultural construct.[547] Aristides' approach to medicine and his perception of his illness were, to a large extent, a 'product of their time'. As alien as a modern reader may find it, Aristides' understanding of his illness as a 'deeply significant life-event, integral to the sufferer's whole being, spiritual, moral and physical',[548] was the commonly held view of illness in the western world from antiquity until the nineteenth century. Therefore Aristides' testimony in the *Sacred Tales* embodies what was likely to have been a typical experience of being ill during the high empire. From his comprehension of his illness, to his choice of whom to consult and whom to address by a prayer, Aristides' narrative of falling ill offers an illuminating picture of the Graeco-Roman health-care system at this time.

543 Gal. 6.836–880 K.
544 Gal. 7.1–41 K.
545 Gal. 7.42–84 K.
546 Gal. 7.85–146 K.
547 See above, pp. 40–44.
548 Porter (1987) 25.

CHAPTER THREE

RECONSIDERING PRIVATE RELIGIONS; RELIGION AND RELIGIOUS EXPERIENCE IN THE *SACRED TALES* OF AELIUS ARISTIDES

Introduction

The *Sacred Tales* are first and foremost a record of religious devotion. They document Aristides' relationship with Asclepius over a time span of three decades, in which the god saved him from the grip of disease, trained him as an orator and generally reinvigorated his will to live. Scholarship of Graeco-Roman religion has historically viewed the *Sacred Tales* as epitomising some fundamental changes in the religious climate.[1] Aristides' devotion to Asclepius has been viewed as part of a general growth in private religions, which coincided with a noticeable decline in the appeal of state religion.[2] Furthermore, the religious meaning of the events Aristides recorded in the *Sacred Tales* has been interpreted by some prominent scholars as an expression of anxiety, typical of their age.[3]

I wish to revisit these claims by questioning to what extent Aristides' religious habits and beliefs were really innovative and eccentric, or whether they were instead shaped by pre-existing and pre-eminent Graeco-Roman traditions. In the first section I will review Aristides' general knowledge of theology by looking at his ideas about the nature of the gods; the form of the Greek pantheon; the inclination of the gods to help mankind; and the means by which Aristides believed mankind could invoke the gods. The

[1] Dodds (1965) 40–44; Festugiére (1954) 85–104; Lane Fox (1986) 160ff.; Liebeschuetz (2000) 1004.

[2] Scholars who accept the distinction between private and public religions view the second century CE as a turning point in the history of religious beliefs and cultic habits, which manifested itself in the form of a shift from communicating with the god through public institutions such as a college of priests or a temple based oracle to a more direct approach; North (1990). Healing cults, according to Liebeschuetz (2000) 1004, provide an excellent example of this tendency. I discuss further some aspects of the religious climate under Marcus' reign in Israelowich (2008).

[3] The term was famously coined by W.H. Auden and applied by his friend Eric R. Dodds (1965) to this period of Roman history.

second section will consider the myth of Asclepius. Thirdly, I will discuss the place of divination in Aristides' religious beliefs. Finally, I will examine the role of culture and society in moulding Aristides' theology, religious habits and beliefs into their particular form.[4] I will identify the agents of culture in society, such as visual images with religious content in art and architecture, as well as social institutions such as temples, festivals and cult, which shaped the religious discourse. I will then assess the degree to which Aristides' beliefs and religious habits were a result of the influence of his environment.

A study of Aristides' theological thought must initially address some issues of methodology and source criticism. Though most of Aristides' corpus of work includes discernible religious themes, the different works within it are of various genres, which means that they cannot all be approached as source material in the same manner. To begin with, Aristides' lectures on theology in his epideictic orations and in his prose hymns were not written or delivered as 'academic' lectures, but as public displays of rhetorical skill. Their content should, therefore, not be taken as Aristides' genuine thoughts or beliefs, but merely as a reworking of ideas that Aristides was familiar with; ideas that he thought his audience expected to hear.[5] On the other hand, the evidence for Aristides' religious cultic habits and beliefs, which can be drawn from the *Sacred Tales*, provides a much better indication of his genuine feelings. Though they were never intended to act as a private account, the *Sacred Tales* contain no general lectures about theology.[6] They concentrate on particular events in which religious beliefs were translated into actions, such as cult, interpretation of dreams, religiously motivated cleansing and journeys of pilgrimage.[7] The evidence from the epideictic orations and from the hymns will, therefore, only be

---

[4] There has been a long-lasting disagreement amongst classicists concerning the use of the term 'belief' to describe pagan religions. I take belief to mean the mental intention which motivates all religious cults. In this respect, I see no reason to limit the use of the term belief solely to Christians and Jews.

[5] Lectures (*dialexeis*) and declamations (*meletai*) which were delivered by the so-called sophists are among the most important phenomena of Greek culture during the high empire; Bowie (2000) 900. These rhetors displayed their skills publicly or as teachers of rhetoric by exercising their perfect command in the Attic dialect of Greek and speaking of a well-known subject from the Greek *paideia*. Their performance was measured according to their ability to master a technique and employ classical themes.

[6] Petsalis-Diomiidis (2010) 124 who rightfully criticized Swain (1996) 255, and Cox-Miller (1994) 204.

[7] Petsalis-Diomidis (2008) argued that if seen through the prism of the *Sacred Tales*, it is possible to find traces of Aristides' profound religious outlook throughout his work.

used for the purpose of forming a picture of the common ideological beliefs which existed at this time and which Aristides alludes to, or presupposes, in his public declamations. Only after identifying these theological ideas in Aristides' private life, as they are portrayed in the *Sacred Tales*,[8] can these religious themes be seen as indicative of his own religious sentiments.

An examination of the formative role of culture and society in shaping Aristides' religious habits and beliefs into their particular form also poses some methodological difficulties in measuring and quantifying such an influence.[9] I shall try to identify the agents who were responsible for teaching the myth of Asclepius and the praxis of his cult and trace their teachings in the *Sacred Tales*. Initially the myth of Asclepius itself has to be examined in order to learn whether Aristides' beliefs and their translation into cultic habits and actions were in accordance with Graeco-Roman traditions. In other words, I will be interested in learning whether Aristides' choice of worshipping Asclepius and of seeking his help after falling ill was normative or subversive.[10] Secondly, the *modus operandi* of the various agents of culture who were teaching this myth needs to be identified and the influence of these agents on Aristides will have to be acknowledged and evaluated. Such agents are, in addition to the Greek canonical authors, classical visual culture and religious festivals, games and the cultic habits in the temples of Asclepius themselves and elsewhere.

One additional issue that needs to be taken into consideration is the role of narrative and narratology in shaping Aristides' portrayal of his religious life. There are two branches of the study of narrative and narratology. One looks at the story as signified ('what happened') and the other looks at the

[8] The *Sacred Tales* were written to be published but are qualitatively different from and of a more personal nature than his orations. See chapter 1.

[9] The general question of the relations between private knowledge, memories and meaningful experiences and public institutions has stood at the heart of some of the most important philosophical investigations of modern times, with repercussions in social sciences (cf. sociology and anthropology). In its broader form, the possibility of a private language was convincingly refuted initially by Wittgenstein and later by various other analytical philosophers, notably S. Kripke, *Wittgenstein: On Rules and Private Language*, and various works of H. Putnam. In the field of anthropology, the ground-breaking work of M. Halbwachs, *On Collective Memory*, demonstrated that human memory can only function within a collective context. In the present context it is enough to note that the examination of the formative role of public institutions on the religious experience of Aristides is an examination of dialectic relationship and that the overall argument presented here borrows from these works of Wittgenstein and Halbwachs. Cf. above, p. 3, n. 6.

[10] I have already looked into this matter in the second chapter, but focused on the medical aspects of Aristides' choice. In this chapter I will focus on the religious aspect of Aristides' devotion to Asclepius.

narrative as a signifier ('the way it is told').[11] Aristides' choices in telling his story and of what to include in the narrative of his religious experience in the *Sacred Tales* (deliberations which he shared with his readership) as well as decisions regarding genre and form of narrative (here too, Aristides made the motivations behind his choices known to his readers) are inseparable from his religious experience because the events that he recorded as well as the act of narrating itself were of religious meaning to Aristides. As discussed above,[12] both aspects of the *Sacred Tales*' narrative, namely their function as a record of events, as well as their religiously-oriented mode of story-telling, were explicitly presented by Aristides as essential aspects of his religious experience.

1. Theology

In early February 149 CE, in an unsuccessful attempt to sail from Clazomenae to Phocaea,[13] Aristides was nearly shipwrecked in a storm. Back at Smyrna, in payment of vows he then made, the oration *Regarding Zeus* was delivered. It is the most detailed exposition of theological thought that we find in Aristides' work. The picture Aristides depicts here of Zeus as the supreme deity who delegates his authority to the other members of the Hellenic pantheon owes much to Plato, the Stoics, and the Orphics.[14] With traditional Greek typology Aristides refers to Zeus as the father of the universe:

> Ζεὺς τὰ πάντα ἐποίησε καὶ Διός ἐστιν ἔργα ὅσα ἐστὶ πάντα, καὶ ποταμοὶ καὶ γῆ καὶ θάλαττα καὶ οὐρανὸς καὶ ὅσα τούτων μεταξὺ ἄνω καὶ ὅσα ὑπὸ ταῦτα, καὶ θεοὶ καὶ ἄνθρωποι καὶ ὅσα ψυχὴν ἔχει καὶ ὅσα εἰς ὄψιν ἀφικνεῖται καὶ ὅσα δεῖ νοήσει λαβεῖν.[15]
>
> Zeus created everything and all that exists is the work of Zeus, rivers, earth, sea, heaven, and that in between these, and all that is above these and all that is beneath, and gods and men, and all that has a soul, and all that is visible, and all that is only conceivable.

---

[11] Seminal here are White (1980) 6, with reference to A. de Tocqueville, *Democracy in America*; J.C. Burckhardt, *The Civilization of the Renaissance in Italy*; J. Huizinga, *The Waning of the Middle Ages*; F. Braudel, *The Mediterranean and the Mediterranean World in the Age of Philip II*. Also valuable is White (1984) and Lévi-Strauss (1966) who discuss the explanatory limitations of historiography in a narrative form.

[12] Chapter one, 'Aelius Aristides and the *Sacred Tales*'.

[13] Aristides discussed the circumstances of this journey in the second *Sacred Tale* (48.12 K). For a study of this journey see Rutherford (1999); Petsalis-Diomidis (2005).

[14] Behr (1968) 72–73, 151–152.

[15] Aristid. *Or.* 43.7 K.

Initially, Aristides says, Zeus had created himself, which leads the author to discuss other traditions of creation, all taken from Greek culture.[16] Zeus was also the creator of time,[17] a theme that could have found its origin in Plato's *Timaeus* and certainly lay at the heart of Greek thinking.

Myths of creation were a common theme in Greek literature, and Aristides' speech brings to mind earlier works.[18] Aristides' *Regarding Zeus* did not aim to introduce a new cosmology. Its merits were in form and grace of presentation. Ideas such as: ἀέρα τε ὑπὲρ ἀμφοτέρων ἔστησε, γῆς καὶ θαλάττης ἀναπνοήν. καὶ πῦρ ἄνωθεν, ὃ δὴ αἰθέρα ὀνομάζουσιν, ἐπιστήσας, τετάρτῳ τούτῳ τὰ πάντα κατέλαβε('he [i.e. Zeus] set the air above both [i.e. air and sea] as means of respiration for the air and the sea, and above all that fire, which we call ether, and he held the universe together with this fourth element') are reminiscent of familiar Greek works.[19] According to Aristides, the world Zeus created was begotten by Love and Necessity, an idea which has some traces in Plato's *Symposium*.[20] Aristides continues and says that when people built cities they dedicated the acropolis to Zeus to imitate the universe.[21] Zeus was also the creator of Law, which he sent with Reverence and Justice,[22] a theme Aristides reiterated in his encomium to Athena.[23] This leads Aristides to one practical point: if Zeus is the creator of mankind and of law he must also be its protector.[24] In stating this Aristides brings to mind the position of Plutarch and other contemporary authors who stressed the positive attributes of god and therefore rejected any need to fear him.[25] Zeus, Aristides explained, is a benefactor and guardian for mankind.[26]

---

16 Aristid. *Or.* 43.8 K.

17 Aristides, *Or.* 43.9 K.

18 With Aristid. *Or.* 43.10 K cf. Hes. *Op.* 19; *Theog.* 728; Arist. *Mete.* b 1.353 a 35f.

19 With Aristid. *Or.* 43.13 K cf. Diog. Laert. 7.137.

20 Ἔρωτά τε καὶ Ἀνάγκην, δύο τούτω συναγωγοτάτω τε καὶ ἰσχυροτάτω, ἐν τοῖς πρῶτα ἐγέννησεν, ὅπως αὐτῷ τὰ πάντα συνέχοιεν. (First of all he begot Love and Necessity, these two powers which are most unifying and most strong, so that they might hold the universe together for him). Aristid. *Or.* 43. 16 K. The antiquity of Eros is asserted in Pl. *Symp* 195b, (and 191d). The meaning of necessity (ἀνάγκη) as law of nature is already attested in Lys. 104.2; Aesch. *Ag.* 725; Pl. *Rep.* 458d.

21 Aristid. *Or.* 1.14–16 L-B. The resemblance between a city and the cosmos is also the subject of D.Chr. *Borysthenitic Oration*,36.31–32.

22 Aristid. *Or.* 43.20 K. This point has also been made before cf. Pl. *Prt.* 322c.

23 Aristid. *Or.* 37.7 K.

24 Aristid. *Or.* 43.22 K.

25 This is the argument presented by Plutarch in his Plut. *De Superst.* for the evolution of the term *superstitio* in the Latin speaking world Grodzynski (1974) is seminal.

26 Aristid. *Or.* 43. 26 K.

Asclepius, being an offspring of Zeus, is also well-disposed towards mankind, and has bestowed upon men the greatest and most universal of benefactions: eternal life through succession, marriage, the begetting of children and the means and recourse of nurture.[27]

Aristides' gods were also responsible for the present form of the cosmos. Zeus himself organised and distributed the functions of the constellation to illuminate the universe

> καὶ ἡ ἡλίου τε ἄπαυστος κίνησις ὑπὲρ γῆς τε καὶ ὑπὸ γῆν Διός ἐστι πρόρρησις ἡλίῳ προειρημένη ὑπὲρ τῆς τοῦ παντὸς κόσμου φανότητος, καὶ σελήνης δρόμοι καὶ χορεῖαι πάντων ἄστρων Διός ἐστι διάκοσμος.[28]

> And the ceaseless motion of the sun above and beneath the earth represents the proclamation of Zeus which he made to the sun concerning the illumination of the whole Universe, and of course the moon and the dances of all the stars are the arrangements of Zeus.

Cosmology, for Aristides, was intrinsically associated with theogony (i.e. genealogy of the gods), which led Aristides to narrate the creation of the rest of the gods by Zeus:

> καὶ Ἀπόλλων ἀνθρώποις χρησμῳδεῖ Διὸς νημερτέα βουλήν, καὶ Ἀσκληπιὸς ἰᾶται, Ἀθηνᾶ τε Ἐργάνη Διὸς γνώμῃ ταύτην εἴληχε τὴν τάξιν, καὶ Ἥρα γαμηλία, καὶ Ἄρτεμις λοχία καὶ κυνηγέτις εὐεργετοῦσιν ἀνθρώπους, τὴν τοῦ μεγάλου σώζουσαι πάντων εὐεργέτου γνώμην. Πᾶνές τε ὀρῶν ἔνοικοι καὶ Νύμφαι ναμάτων ἐπίσκοποι σὺν Διὶ τὴν κληρουχίαν ἔχουσι. Ποσειδῶν τε καὶ Διόσκουροι σώζουσι τοὺς πλέοντας, πειθόμενοι Διί, καὶ Μοῦσαι μουσικὴν εὗρον καὶ κατέδειξαν Διὸς βουληθέντος εἶναι Μούσας καὶ μουσικήν, θεῶν ἅμα καὶ ἀνθρώπων ἕνεκα.[29]

> Apollo gives as oracles to mankind the unerring wish of Zeus. And Asclepius heals assisting Zeus. And Athena of Crafts has been allotted this position by the will of Zeus. And Hera of Marriages and Artemis, both she of Childbirth and the Huntress, benefit mankind in keeping with the will of the great benefactor of all. And the Pans who dwell in the mountains and the Nymphs who watch over the streams hold their allotment with the blessing of Zeus. Obedient to Zeus, Poseidon and the Dioscuri save those at the sea. And the Muses have invented and taught the art of music, since Zeus willed that the Muses and music exist both for the sake of the gods and mankind.

---

[27] Ibid.

[28] Aristid. *Or.* 43.24 K.

[29] Aristid. *Or.* 43.25 K.

In this depiction of the Greek pantheon, it was not necessary for Aristides to choose between the various deities.[30] His allegiances could have been pledged to more than one deity, as was indeed the case.[31]

As an omnipresent deity Zeus' relation with mankind resembles that of a teacher and his pupils.[32] Aristides concludes:

> Ζεὺς πάντων πατὴρ καὶ οὐρανοῦ καὶ γῆς καὶ θεῶν καὶ ἀνθρώπων καὶ ποταμῶν καὶ φυτῶν, καὶ διὰ τοῦτον ὁρῶμεν καὶ ἔχομεν ὁπόσα ἔχομεν. οὗτος ἁπάντων εὐεργέτης καὶ ἔφορος καὶ προστάτης, οὗτος πρύτανις καὶ ἡγεμὼν καὶ ταμίας ὄντων καὶ γιγνομένων ἁπάντων, οὗτος δοτὴρ ἁπάντων, οὗτος ποιητής.[33]
>
> Zeus is the father of all, rivers, heaven, earth, gods, mankind, animals, and plants. And through him we see and have all that we have. He is the benefactor, overseer, and patron of all. He is the president, governor, and steward of all being and of all things coming into being. He is the giver of all things, he is the creator of all things.

However it was Asclepius who was the focus of Aristides' religious devotion, no doubt due to his own fragile health. Aristides delivered his encomium *To Asclepius* in the temple of Zeus-Asclepius at Pergamum, perhaps on January 6, 177 CE, at the celebration of the Night Festival.[34] The speech includes a vivid description of the present-day cult of Asclepius in the Asclepieion, providing important evidence of the daily prayers and sacrifices.[35] In a manner typical of a Second Sophistic author, Aristides traced the origin of Asclepius' cult back to classical Greece, citing no less an authority than the poet Hesiod to support his claim.[36] Furthermore, Aristides expressed his gratitude to the god through oratory.[37] The emphasis on oratory, which 'seems particularly proper to me' (ἡ δ' ἐπὶ τοῦ λόγου μοι πολὺ δὴ μάλιστα

---

30 Indeed, Lane Fox, referring to the second century CE, commented that 'pagans had never had a wider choice of gods than during this period'. However, Lane-Fox noticed, the 'various cults show no sign of competition for people's sole adherences'. Furthermore, this wide range of pagan cults was not seen as problematic to its pagan worshipper. Among contemporaries, only the Christians found it theologically problematic. Lane-Fox (1986) 34.

31 In the *Sacred Tales* Aristides is portrayed not only as a faithful worshipper of Asclepius, but also of Zeus, Athena, Apollo and Sarapis. Cf. Apollo: Aristid. *Or.* 49.12. Athena: 48.41–44; Zeus: 49.20, 39, 40, 41, 48 K.

32 Aristid. *Or.* 43.26 K.

33 Aristid. *Or.* 43.29 K.

34 Behr Vol. ii (1986) 416.

35 Daily prayers: Aristid. *Or.* 42.1 K; sacrifices: Aristid. *Or.* 42.2 K.

36 Aristid. *Or.* 42.2 following Hes. *Op.* 336: Κὰδ δύναμιν δ' ἔρδειν ἱέρ' ἀθανάτοισι θεοῖσιν 'to sacrifice according to one's means'.

37 Ibid.

προσήκειν φαίνεται),[38] allowed Aristides to achieve two interlinked goals: the first is eulogizing Asclepius by tracing the origin of his cult to the Greek golden age. The second is to glorify himself as an orator, by hinting that he was trained by Asclepius himself.[39]

The speech *To Asclepius* makes some use of the author's private experiences, and Aristides implicitly goes through all the benefactions the god had bestowed upon him throughout his life. However, unlike in the *Sacred Tales*, the narrative of the speech *To Asclepius* is far less personal. Moreover, the author referred his readers back to his *Sacred Tales* for further details, which seemed to him unnecessary in the present context.[40] Indeed, it is only after reading the *Sacred Tales* that the personal experiences of Aristides manifest themselves in this oration.

The overall picture that Aristides portrayed in his public declamations, and which is also indicated in the *Sacred Tales*, is that religion, in its traditional Greek sense, is the foundation of the social order. In tune with one strand of Greek tradition, Aristides put forward the view that the law is both divine and absolute,[41] and he ascribed to Athena the foundation of civil society by establishing cities and laws:

> πρῶτον μὲν γὰρ τῆς ὀρείου καὶ καθ' ἑκάστους διαίτης ἀπαλλαγῆναι καὶ συνελθόντας οἰκεῖν ἐν ταὐτῷ μίαν συνοικίαν κοινὴν περιβαλλομένους ἥδ' ἐστὶν ἡ πείσασα, καὶ εἰσὶν αἱ πόλεις δῶρα 'Αθηνᾶς· ὅθεν δὴ καὶ πολιοῦχος ἅπασι κέκληται. τὰς δὲ ἀκροπόλεις ἐξεῖλον αὐτῇ δικαίως, ἅμα μὲν σύμβολον τῆς γενέσεως, ἅμα δὲ ὥσπερ τοῖς βασιλεῦσι καὶ ἡγεμόσι τεμένη καὶ χώρους ἐξαιροῦσιν, οὕτω τῇ τοῦ παντὸς ἡγησαμένῃ θεῷ τὰ ἐπικαιρότατα ἐξεῖλον. ἓν μὲν δὴ τοῦτο λέγω κοινὸν εὐεργέτημα τῆς θεοῦ, πρὸς τὴν καθ' ἡμέραν δίαιταν, πολιτείαν καὶ νόμους.[42]
>
> First of all it is she who persuaded men to give up their solitary mountain life and to assemble and dwell together in the compass of a single, common

---

[38] Ibid.

[39] This is a seminal theme in the *Sacred Tales*, which were already in circulation by the time the speech *To Asclepius* was delivered. Aristides must have assumed his audience was familiar with this other work of his. See above, pp. 26–29. The connection between these two themes is that Asclepius, so Aristides repeatedly argued in the *Sacred Tales*, encouraged him to resume practising rhetoric while convalescing in his temple and actually trained him and improved his skills.

[40] Cf. Aristid. *Or.* 42.10 K.

[41] The subject of the Greek views of *nomos* is a notoriously complicated matter. The myth of its establishment in Athens which was told, amongst others, by Aeschylus has it that not even the purification rites carried out by Apollo himself are able any longer to drive away the Erinyes from Orestes (Aesch. *Eum.* 276–283). Only a formal juridical verdict (i.e. according to the *nomoi*) is able to do so. For a modern discussion see Parker (1996) 43–55, Lloyd-Jones (1983), and Price (1999) 78–79.

[42] Aristid. *Or.* 37.13 K.

> settlement. And the cities are a gift of Athena, for which reason all men also call her Poliuchus. They have justly set aside their acropolises for her as a token of her birth and at the same time just as they set aside precincts and lands for their emperors and governors, so they have set aside the most important places for the goddess who has governed the universe. I say that this truly is one universal benefit of the goddess for our daily life, government and laws.

The interconnections between theology, cosmology and social order were a common theme during the high empire, both amongst the so-called Second Sophistic authors and beyond.[43] In addition to Aristides, there were other Greek authors of the period, notably Plutarch and Dio of Prusa (two generations earlier) who used religious argumentation and *exempla* to support their own political claims.[44]

To conclude, Aristides' theology was far from eccentric, innovative or subversive. Aristides was aware of the important role of traditional Greek religion in maintaining the existing social order.[45] His lectures on theology are a tribute to Greek *paideia* and a comparison between the contents of his epideictic orations and hymns with his actual religious praxis, as depicted in the *Sacred Tales*, bears no trace of a dichotomy between his public persona and his private life. From his comments on the genealogy of Asclepius,[46] through his consultation with oracles,[47] to the general picture of the Greek pantheon which emerges from the scattered appearances of Zeus, Athena, Apollo and Asclepius, the *Sacred Tales* portray a picture of an attempt to live a traditional Greek religious life.

2. The Myth of Asclepius

Having first set the theological framework in which Aristides experienced religion, I will now provide the context of the Asclepius myth. Aristides devoted the *Sacred Tales* to Asclepius and they record his relationship with the god. I will investigate whether Aristides' devotion to Asclepius and to his cult mirrored the teachings of an age-old Greek tradition, or whether his devotion discloses some traces of theological novelties. This issue is

43 Cf. D.Chr. *Or.* 36.31 with Russell's (1992) commentary ad loc.
44 Sheppard (1984) 238–240.
45 This theme comes to the fore in Aristides' civic orations, when advocating for concord.
46 Aristid. *Or.* 50.39–40 K.
47 Aristid. *Or.* 49.12, 38 K.

of wider importance because the agents of culture who were responsible for the transmission of myth (e.g. Greek literature, temples and cult, religious festivals and the visual culture) also defined Greek identity in general. In consequence, if Aristides' religious beliefs and behaviour, as they are depicted in his *Sacred Tales*, broke with the teachings of Greek tradition this could indicate that the understanding of these myths within Greek culture as a whole had similarly altered in this period. If, however, it becomes evident that the *Sacred Tales* were faithful to the teachings of Greek *paideia*—and that Aristides' religious beliefs and behaviour were consolidated into their particular form due to the indoctrinating influence of the classical authorities—it could support the commonly advocated argument for the prevalence of Greek culture and Greek *paideia* during the high empire on a religious terrain, as well as the cultural one.[48]

Initially, there is a need to look into this myth in some detail in order to establish whether approaching Asclepius would be the obvious course of action for someone who faced the same difficulties and afflictions as Aristides. Furthermore, would he have been expected to seek help from Asclepius in an equivalent manner to Aristides and with similar expectations? It is therefore pertinent to enquire what were the powers the myth ascribed to Asclepius, how should the devout invoke this healing god and how popular was Asclepius' cult during the high empire. The answers to these questions have wider implications. As we shall see, participants in the cult of Asclepius approached their god as individuals, not as part of a collective, which is to be expected in the case of a healing deity. Any general changes of pattern concerning the worship of Asclepius, such as an increase or decrease in the number of the cult's followers, might illuminate broader areas of Graeco-Roman history than simply the private life of Aelius Aristides. From an indication of the general health of the Graeco-Roman world to the level of support for state-organised cult, the religious experience of Aristides can provide a significant contribution to the study of the high empire.

[48] The role of classical Greek culture and the function of *mimesis* in shaping Greek identity during Aristides' lifetime exceed the scope of the present study. Important contributions include Schmid on Atticism (1887–1897); Bowersock's (1969) study of the place of the Greek sophists in their social and political context; Bowie (1970) analysed the dialectic relations between the sophists and their image of Greek past; Swain (1996) looked into some of the main authors of the era and Schmitz (1997) inquired how the monopoly over *paideia* was translated into political power; Whitmarsh (2001) looked into the mechanism of *mimesis* during Aristides' lifetime.

The hero Asclepius, as depicted by Homer in the *Catalogue of Ships*, is the father of Machaon and Podalirius, leaders of men from Tricca, Ithome, and Oechalia.[49] The ancients seemed to have accepted the Homeric claim of Asclepius' origin and it was generally agreed that he belonged to the Homeric age.[50] Asclepius gained his medical knowledge from Chiron,[51] who was not only a friend and patron of heroes but the inventor of herbal medicine as well.[52] Homer's testimony places Machaon, and thereby Asclepius, in Thessaly, which is in agreement with the tradition Homer was likely to have followed. The connection between Asclepius and Chiron, the wise centaur who was skilled in the knowledge of drugs, indicates that Asclepius was a familiar figure in Thessalian mythology.[53] Chiron himself was a Thessalian hero living on Mount Pelion, which was renowned for its herbs.[54] It is more than plausible then that Asclepius originated from the same place.

The proper legend of a hero must give his ancestry, the tale of his birth and his education, his deeds, and his death. In the case of Asclepius, a poem of Pindar is the first instance where all this information is provided coherently, and Asclepius is labelled as a hero.[55] According to Pindar,[56] Asclepius was the son of Apollo and Coronis. His mother, when bearing the child of the god, fell in love with a mortal. When the god came to learn this, he sent Artemis to kill Coronis, but he spared his child and put him under Chiron's care. Asclepius was educated by the sage and grew up to be a great physician. Unfortunately Asclepius was given to unlawful greed; he would cure for money those who were doomed to die.[57] Therefore Zeus, the king of all gods and administrator of justice slew Asclepius with his thunderbolt, thus rightfully punishing a sinner, who was a son of a sinful mother. Such is Pindar's testimony in a poem that has all the attributes of a tragedy: the

49 Hom. *Il.* 2.729–733.

50 Edelstein & Edelstein vol. ii. (1945) 2f.

51 Hom. *Il.* 4.192–219.

52 Edelstein & Edelstein vol. ii (1945) 5. For Chiron in the Roman era cf. Plin. *Nat. Hist.* 7.196: *medicinam Aegyptii apud ipsos volunt repertam, alii per Arabum Babylonis et Apollonis filium, herbariam et medicamentariam a Chirone Saturni et Philyrae filio.* (Medicine according to the Egyptians was discovered among themselves, but according to others through the agency of Arabus son of Babylon and Apollo; and the science of herbs and drugs was discovered by Chiron, the son of Saturn and Philyra).

53 For Asclepius' Thessalian connection Cf. Str. 9.5.17; Hom. *Il.* 2.729–732; *h.Hom.* 16.3; Pind. *Pyth.* 3.34; Currie (2005) 354–355.

54 Edelstein & Edelstein vol. ii (1945) 22.

55 Pind. *Pyth.* 3.1–58.

56 Pind. *Pyth.* 3.8.

57 Pind. *Pyth.* 3.36–37.

descent into crime of successive generations; men who are at the mercy of their passions; who are irreverent toward the gods; and whose fall, therefore, is inevitable.[58]

Pindar's version, however, was not generally accepted in classical antiquity. Instead it is the version we know through the work of Apollodorus the mythographer that gained most credibility.[59] Apollodorus speaks of two genealogies of Asclepius. In both Apollo is the father, but in one account the mother was Arsinoë and in the other it was Coronis. According to Apollodorus the second version (in which Coronis is Asclepius' mother) was only believed by some, but it is the only one of the two traditions Apollodorus gave in full.[60] It was also the version Aristides accepted.[61] According to Apollodorus, Apollo killed Coronis because of her intention to marry Ischys. Coronis' child, Asclepius, was entrusted to Chiron who taught him to hunt and the art of medicine. He became an especially skilled surgeon, but in addition to his medical activities Asclepius was also a sorcerer. Athena had shared with him the blood of the Gorgon, which he used for the benefit of men as well as for their destruction. Consequently, Zeus decided to kill him because he was afraid of humans' losing their fear of death and thus their reverence toward the gods.[62] The Arsinoë version is, most likely, later, and was used to serve political goals of the Messenians after 370 BCE.[63]

In all traditions Apollo is Asclepius' father. It is from Apollo, the old god of medicine, that Asclepius inherited his medical skills. Moreover, although a hero is always associated with a region of origin, the connection of Asclepius

---

58 Bowra (1968) 78.

59 Apollod. *Bibl.* 3.10.3, 5–4,1. The scholiast on Pind. *Pyth.* 3.14 quotes authorities on both sides. Asclepiades and an Argive author by the name of Socrates championed Arsinoë. These authors' support of the Arsinoë verion, seeing in the god and his sons their fellow countrymen, is to be expected from authors with a strong regional sense of identity, cf. Paus. 2.26.3–7; 4.3.2; 4.31.12. On the other side there is a long tradition supporting Coronis, cf. *h.Hom.* 16; Pind. *Pyth.* 1.14 ff.; Ap. Rhod. 4.616 ff.; Diod. Sic. 4.71.1; 5.74.6; Paus. 2.26.3–7; Hyg. *Fab.* 202; id. *Astronom.* 2.40; Servius, on Virgil, *Aen.* 4.617; Lactantius Placidus, on Statius, *Theb.* 3.506; *Scriptores rerum mythicarum Latini*, ed. G.H. Bode, vol. i. 17, 37. J.G. Frazer referred to Apollodorus' version as 'an accurate record of what the Greeks in general believed'. Cf. Frazer's introduction to his edition of Apollodorus work, p. XVII (Loeb).

60 A Xanthian inscription from the third century BC, from the temple of Leto at Xanthus in Lycia also named Coronis as Ascplepius' mother. Cf. *SEG* 38.1476, with Cameron (2004) 224–225.

61 Aristid. *Or.* 47.73 K.

62 Apollod. *Bibl.* 3.10.4 (passage's authenticity is defended by Cameron (2004) 100–101): this story is reiterated by Zenobius, *Cent.* 1.18. Diod. Sic. 4.71.1–3 has it that Asclepius' exceptional skills as a physician actually changed the death rate. This upset Hades, who in return complained to Zeus, who then killed Asclepius with a thunderbolt.

63 Cf. Paus. 2.26.7.

with Apollo (unlike his mortal mother) gained him pan-Hellenic recognition. It was Apollo who entrusted Asclepius to the hands of Chiron, thus designating his destiny.[64] Pindar says so explicitly.[65] The hero was not merely descended from Apollo, the physician, he was designated to follow his father's path.[66] Yet unlike most other heroes there are only few indicators of his character: no love affairs, tales of friendship or hatred, or accounts of rivalry or quarrel with men or gods are attached to him. Asclepius is one of the least humanised of all the Greek heroes.[67] All his being is integrated into the one function of healing.

Unlike Asclepius the hero who had vanished and lived only in the memory of men full of admiration, Asclepius the immortal god was very much alive in his shrines such as those in Epidaurus, Cos, Tricca, Athens and Pergamum.[68] The first testimony we have of Asclepius the god is an Athenian inscription from 420 BCE recording the god's arrival at the city.[69] Asclepius must have been recognised as a deity in Epidaurus before this date, as it was from Epidaurus that he came to Athens.[70] Yet for Pindar, writing in c. 475 BCE, Asclepius was a hero not a god. It is therefore suggested that the chthonian Asclepius was first venerated only in an isolated part of Greece, in Thessaly, where Tricca was presumably the oldest place of the cult,[71] but by the fifth century BCE Asclepius was already pan-Hellenic.[72] However, as late as Aristides' day, when Pausanias arrived in Epidaurus he learned that Coronis, the god's mother, came to this land to give birth to Asclepius, a testimony to an on-going and still vibrant local tradition.[73]

The oldest divine birth-myth attested is found in the Homeric hymn to Asclepius.[74] Here the god is the son of Apollo and Coronis, the daughter of

---

64 Pherecydes' transcription of the Hesiodic poem = *Scholia in Pindarum*, *Pyth.* 3.59. The most recent collection of the fragments of Pherecydes Atheniensis = *FGrHist* 3 is Fowler (2000) 272–364.

65 Pind. *Pyth.* 3.45–46.

66 Edelstein & Edelstein vol. ii. (1945) 38.

67 Edelstein & Edelstein vol. ii. (1945) 53.

68 For a history of the Asclepieion in Cos see Sherwin-White (1978) 98, 173, 334–346; for the Asclepieion in Athens see Parker (1996) 179–181; Epidaurus: LiDonnici (1995), Tomlinson (1983) 21–33 and Burford (1969) 13–24; Pergamum: Radt (1988) 250–271, Petsalis-Diomidis (2010).

69 *IG*, II^2 4960a.

70 On the Athenian Asclepieion see Aleshire (1989).

71 Edelstein & Edelstein vol. ii. (1945) 65; Parker (1996) 179–182.

72 Currie (2005) 355.

73 Paus. 2.26.3–5.

74 Ἰητῆρα νόσων Ἀσκληπιὸν ἄρχομ' ἀείδειν / υἱὸν Ἀπόλλωνος τὸν ἐγείνατο δῖα Κορωνὶς / Δωτίῳ

Phlegyas who was born in the Dotian plain. The hymn is in perfect agreement with the Hesiodic narrative except that all aspects of violence are excluded. Here Coronis gives birth naturally to Asclepius, unlike the heroic version of a forced caesarean operation.[75] It is the story of the birth of a god that is being told here, with the influence of Delphi in producing this particular narrative.[76] Furthermore, the tradition of the Homeric hymns lasted throughout antiquity with only one change: Asclepius lost his affiliation with Thessaly.

The myth of Asclepius the god was a deification of the heroic saga.[77] Yet, as Edelstein and Edelstein have noted,[78] for an appreciation of the god Asclepius it is not enough to say that he was a deified hero. The questions of what were his powers, were they limited to the healing of men, and was this restricted jurisdiction a result of the god's own discretion, need to be addressed. We know that in polytheistic theology not all gods were equal and therefore it is important to ask where Asclepius stood in this hierarchy. It appears from the ancient sources that Asclepius was 'the one who gently takes pains with the sick'.[79] His very name came to represent the standard of medical care.[80] Asclepius was also perceived as protector from ailments.[81] He stood for the perfect application of the medical art. Bearing in mind that those arriving in the Asclepieia had already been dismissed by physicians as 'hopeless cases'[82] the pressing need for a deity of this kind becomes clear.

However, Asclepius was never seen as a god of the first rank. He was late to have become a deity, which led some to question his status as a god.[83]

ἐν πεδίῳ κούρῃ Φλεγύου βασιλῆος, / χάρμα μέγ' ἀνθρώποισι, κακῶν θελκτῆρ' ὀδυνάων. / Καὶ σὺ μὲν οὕτω χαῖρε ἄναξ· λίτομαι δέ σ' ἀοιδῇ.

'For Asclepius the healer of sickness first I sing, son of Apollo, born in the Dotian Plain to the lady Coronis, daughter of king Phlegyas, a great joy to mankind, the soother of horrid pains. So I salute you, lord; I supplicate you with my song' [trans. West (2003)]. Hom. *Hymni*, 16.

75 Edelstein & Edelstein vol. ii (1945) 68.

76 Nock (1933) 23 argued that the Homeric hymns were composed in the interests of those cults with which Delphi identified itself.

77 Edelstein & Edelstein vol. ii (1945) 76; Currie (2005) 355.

78 Edelstein & Edelstein vol. ii (1945) 81.

79 Eust. *Il.* 4.202.

80 Cf. Hippoc. *Ep.* 2; Gal. *De Sanitate Tuenda*, 1.12.15; D.Chr. *Or.* 6.23–24; Crin. *Epigrammata*, 6; Gow-Page; Ath. 1.51.28e; 10.44.434d; Max. Tyr. 5.4 f.; 14.8g; 36.5 f.; 40.3d–e; Nicephoros Gregoras, *Byzantinae Historiae*, 26.20.

81 Porph. *Quaestiones Homericae*, a, 68; Scholia in Lycophronem, *Ad Alexandram*, 1054; Eudocia Augusta, *Violarium*, 11.

82 Cf. Aristides himself.

83 Late arrival at the pantheon: Cic. *Nat. D.*, 3.15.39; Arn. *Adv. Nat.* 3.39; Lucian, *Iupp. Trag.* 21; Asclepius' divine status has been questioned by a Christian: Justin, *Apol.* 25. 1.

For Maximus Tyrius Asclepius was evidently not an equal of the Olympians: 'And it is doubtless through the possession of emotion that the god is inferior to the rest of the *daimons*.[84] For what their natural characteristics were when they dwelt on earth, these they do not desire wholly to relinquish'.[85] A century before Maximus Tyrius, Dionysius of Halicarnassus was clear in his distinction between the twelve prominent gods, the lesser gods, and the demigods to whom Asclepius belonged.[86] In a division between celestial and earthly gods Asclepius belonged to the latter.[87]

As a god Asclepius healed those who were willing to be his patients in his sanctuaries.[88] There the divine healer performed miracles.[89] The ailments he had treated disappeared during a night of incubation. In oracles and dreams he prescribed treatment and drugs. The foundation of the Asclepieia naturally set up a special relation between certain places and the god. The Epidaurian Isyllus, for example, saw his god bear arms to aid the Lacedaemonians, and the Spartans were convinced by Isyllus and saw in Asclepius their saviour.[90] This episode, however, was the only grand scale public benefaction of Asclepius.[91] Usually his benefactions to society were lower key: important documents were entrusted to his temple,[92] and the dignity of a community was increased by the function of his shrine as an asylum.[93]

During Aristides' lifetime Asclepius was perceived as a moral deity, treating only those he saw fit to be saved, and training his followers in a philosophic life. It is of no surprise then that on the entrance of the Epidaurus' Asclepieion was inscribed: 'pure must be he who enters the fragrant temple; purity means to think nothing but holy thoughts'.[94] The healing process was to induce moral improvement as well: *Bonus intra, melius exi*.[95] Aristides

---

84 Maximus held the major Olympians to be *daimones* too, not just Asclepius, Cf. Max. Tyr. 8.5–6.

85 Καὶ τοῦτό ἐστιν ἀμέλει τὸ ἐμπαθές, ᾧ ἐλαττοῦται δαίμων θεοῦ. Ὡς γὰρ εἶχον φύσεως, ὅτε περὶ γῆν ἦσαν, οὐκ ἐθέλουσιν ταύτης παντάπασιν ἀπαλλάττεσθαι. Max. Tyr. 9.7. a-i.

86 Dion. Hal. *Ant. Rom.* 7.72.13.

87 Artem. 2. 34.

88 Edelstein & Edelstein vol. ii (1945) 101.

89 One of the most detailed sources for these miraculous acts of divine grace is, of course, Aristides' own *Sacred Tales*.

90 *IG* IV^2 1 128, v, 57–79. See discussion in Furley and Bremer vo. i. (2001) 227–240 and vol. ii. (2001) 180–192.

91 Edelstein & Edelstein vol. ii (1945) 103.

92 *Iscr. Di Cos* ED 14.

93 Tac. *Ann.* 4.14.1–2.

94 ἁγνὸν χρὴ ωαοῖο θυώδεος ἐντὸς ἰόντα / ἔμμεναι, ἁγνεία δ' ἐστὶ φρονεῖν ὅσια. Quoted by Porph. *Abst.* 2. 19.

95 *CIL* VIII 1. 2584.

explicitly said that if the god [i.e. Asclepius] were unwilling to help him it would have meant that the god did not see him fit to live.[96] Artemidorus, a contemporary of Aristides, noted that the meaning of Asclepius in a dream is that of a true judge of life and death.[97]

Most of Asclepius' worshippers were sick themselves, and the simplest way of approaching the deity was through prayer.[98] Yet although Asclepius often gave help after prayer alone, the most effective way to receive healing was through dreams in his sanctuaries.[99] Before approaching Asclepius in his temple the sick had to perform preliminary rites of purification.[100] When the patient was healed he was obliged to fulfil his vows.[101] In the Asclepieia the god was honoured with regular sacrifices, which rested in the hands of the priests.[102] When performing cult the priests were usually clad in white—in Pergamum they wore a purple robe[103] and Egyptian shoes[104]—and their hair was bound with a white fillet,[105] all of which added a distinctive visual character to the religious ceremony.[106] In addition to the regular services, Asclepius was worshipped with celebrations that recurred at certain intervals and to which people came from near and far.[107] These religious ceremonies surely also had a powerful and educational effect on the participants. In addition, on every occasion in which Asclepius' cult was practised, it was accompanied by singing and hymns which conveyed contents taken from the myth.[108] Another equally effective aspect of Asclepius' cult was the games which were connected to many of the festivals.[109]

Asclepius was also the patron and the saviour of the family, as is evident from Aristides.[110] His jurisdiction was not restricted to medicine *per se*. Moreover, as a patron of medicine Asclepius also gave oracles and, because

---

96 Aristid. *Or.* 28.132 K.
97 Artem. 5. 13.
98 E.g. Marinus, *Vita Procli*, Cp. 31.
99 Edelstein & Edelstein, Vol. ii (1945) 186.
100 *I. Perg.* II. 264 = *SEG* 4.681; *IG* IV^2 1. 121. 5.
101 *IG* IV^2 1. 5; Ael. *Fragmenta*, 101.
102 Cf. *I. Perg.* II. 251; *IG* II^2 1163.
103 Ps. Aristid. *Or.* 30.27 K.
104 Aristid. *Or.* 47.61 K.
105 Ov. *Met.* 15. 676.
106 It is, however, noteworthy that these items were not mentioned in the Pergamene *lex sacra*; the text was published and edited by Wörle (1969), and later by Petsalis-Diomidis (2010) 224–226.
107 Edelstein & Edelstein, Vol. ii (1945) 195–199.
108 Edelstein & Edelstein, Vol. ii (1945) 199–208.
109 Edelstein & Edelstein, Vol. ii (1945) 208–213.
110 Aristid. *Or.* 42.5 K.

medicine and mantic were closely connected, physicians who demonstrated their skill by accurate prognosis were often taken as soothsayers.[111] Epidaurian inscriptions show that Asclepius' oracular power went beyond the realm of medicine,[112] and this quality of the deity is well attested in Aristides' *Sacred Tales* and in the work of Lucian.[113] The Christian author Origen, in his polemic treatise *Contra Celsum*, stated that Celsus was also acquainted with the reputation of the Asclepieia as centres of oracles.[114] Later Christian authors frowned upon the habit of incubation in a quest for prophetic dreams, dismissing it as a Jewish habit.[115] It thus appears that the image of Asclepius, and the nature of his relationship with his worshippers that Aristides depicted, reflected widespread trends in classical antiquity. Asclepius was the plausible and natural choice of an educated Greek (and Roman) struck by disease during the high empire.

The role of protector of medicine assigned to Asclepius an essential position in the picture of the cosmos. Asclepius was thought to hold responsibility over the health of the universe; he was the world's physician.[116] For Aristides it was Asclepius who 'guides and regulates the universe, the saviour of the world, and the guardian of the immortal ... he who saves that which always exists and that which is in the state of becoming' (οὗτός ἐσθ' ὁ τὸ πᾶν ἄγων καὶ νέμων σωτὴρ τῶν ὅλων καὶ φύλαξ τῶν ἀθανάτων, εἰ δὲ θέλεις τραγικώτερον εἰπεῖν, ἔφορος οἰάκων, σώζων τά τε ὄντα ἀεὶ καὶ τὰ γιγνόμενα).[117] Such philosophical ideas were common in Aristides' day,[118] and Edelstein and Edelstein are surely correct in objecting to André Boulanger's view that Aristides voiced his own thoughts on the matter. Aristides, the Edelsteins noted, was not a metaphysician. On the rare occasions where issues of a speculative nature are discussed he echoed the main trains of thought of the time.[119] Asclepius revealed to Aristides that he was 'the soul of the

[111] E.g. Philostr. *VA* 3. 44. As has been said before, even the great Galen was often seen as a magician when procuring accurate prognosis cf. Gal. *Prog*. 14. 601 K = *CMG* 5.8.1.

[112] *IG*, IV^2 1. 121–122, 127.

[113] In addition to the numerous examples from the *Sacred Tales*, Aristides reiterated this claim in his hymn to Asclepius: *Or*. 42.5 K; see also Lucian, *Deor. Cons*. 16.

[114] Origen, *C. Cels*. 3.3.

[115] Cf. Jerome's translation of Eusebius, *In Isiam Commentaria*, 18. 65.

[116] Edelstein & Edelstein vol. ii. (1945)106.

[117] Aristid. *Or*. 42.4 K. One should, however, bear in mind that at least some of these descriptions were a matter of literary convention.

[118] The Platonist school regained its position as the most popular of all four philosophical schools during Aristides' lifetime (Russell [1973] 73). For an authoritative and concise discussion of the various Platonic views of this age see Dillon (1977).

[119] Boulanger (1923) 199; Edelstein and Edelstein vol. ii (1945) 107 n. 21.

universe',[120] which was a seminal theme in Platonic and Neo-Platonic thought, dating back to Plato's *Timaeus* 34b.[121] For Julian the Apostate, Asclepius was the keeper of the safety of the world;[122] it is through him that the elements do not loosen their indestructible bond; it is through him that the universe remains young and healthy.[123] The only difference between the image of Asclepius as it appears in Aristides' *Sacred Tales* and as it appears in the works of (Neo)-Platonic philosophers is the absence of personal involvement. From a philosophical point of view, Aristides conceived of Asclepius just as the Platonists did.

The myth of Asclepius and the myth's diffusion sets the context for many of the religious experiences Aristides recorded in his *Sacred Tales*. As demonstrated above, Aristides turned to Asclepius in pursuit of health-care. His appeals to the god were mediated by the medical and priestly establishments.[124] Acquaintance with the myth of Asclepius, its popularity and the common patterns of its cult not only explains why Aristides turned to Asclepius after falling ill. It also discloses why Aristides chose to convalesce in the Pergamene Asclepieion; why he believed that Asclepius revealed himself to him in his dreams and in other ways; and even why he thought that the synergy between physicians and priests, which is one of the most remarkable themes of the *Sacred Tales*, is not just possible but also natural and desirable. Although the cult of Asclepius is one of the so-called personal religions—a generic name for all cults which the worshipper approached as an individual—it seems that Aristides' inclination to worship Asclepius was not an act of religious dissent or a sign of a general cultural change. On the contrary, for Aristides it was a choice of Greekness.

3. Divination, Oracles and Dreams

Perhaps the most compelling argument for describing the religious experience of Aristides as personal or private is the abundance of occurrences where Aristides communicated directly with a deity. Divination, either by

120 οὗτος δή σοί ἐστιν ὃν καλεῖ Πλάτων τοῦ παντὸς ψυχήν. ἀναβλέπω τε δὴ καὶ ὁρῶ Ἀσκληπιὸν τὸν ἐν Περγάμῳ ἐνιδρυμένον ἐν τῷ οὐρανῷ. Aristid. *Or.* 50.56 K.

121 Pl. *Tim.* 34b. For the prevalence of this theme of the world's soul amongst middle-Platonists cf. Dillon (1977) 45–46, 82, 217, 252, 282–284, 287, 289, 356, 394–395.

122 Julian *In Helium Regem*, 153b.

123 Sallustius (4th c. CE) *De Dis*, 6.

124 Examples for such mediation are the instances in which Aristides consulted physicians and priests concerning the true meaning of his dreams and the support both physicians and priests bestowed upon him when taking Asclepius' advice.

oracles, dreams or visions was a way for the gods to divulge valuable information to Aristides about his health and what he should do to improve it; about the present and about the future; and about his relationships with others, usually without the need of an intermediary. Aristides himself was keen to acknowledge the content of his dreams, his visions, the voices he heard and the messages he received from oracles as divine words. A number of questions arise from Aristides' experiences. How common were such divine interventions in human lives in Aristides' world? In what fashion were they executed? How was one to know whether it was the god who sent a message? Was there a need for interpretation of the god's transmission, and, if so, who was qualified to perform such an act? What was the role of society and culture in teaching its members how to identify the god's word, how to invoke and communicate with a deity and who to turn to when assistance was needed? In this section I look into the role of divination, oracles and dreams in the religious experience of Aristides with an attempt to place this experience of an individual in a wider social context. Specifically I will consider whether Aristides' acquired his understanding of these notions from the world around him.

Divination in the Graeco-Roman world meant a divinely inspired pronouncement concerning the future in consort with a divine power and it was a seminal aspect of religious life in classical antiquity.[125] Auguste Bouché-Leclerq defined his subject matter in his influential and still highly relevant *Histoire de la divination dans l'antiquité*, as:

> La divination est la produit d'une idée religieuse qui a, de tout temps, possédé la conscience humaine, la foi en la Providence. Elle ne présuppose que les deux conditions ou postulats dont la réunion constitue le fond de toute doctrine religieuse, à savoir, l'existence d'une divinité intelligente et la possibilité de rapports réciproques entre l'homme et la divinité; et elle en est

[125] An interesting introduction to the meaning and use of divination in the various Greek philosophical schools during the high empire is Ps. Plut. *Placita Philosophorum* 5.1 [ed. Mau (1971) p. 133]. Interestingly, after looking into divination, the author then moves on to discuss the formation of dreams (ibid.). For modern scholarship on divination in the Greek world see: Flacelière (1976). On sacrificial divination: van Straten (1988), 51–68; Jameson (1986), 59–66; Burkert examined the origin of this habit in his: *The Orientalizing Revolution* (1992), 41–53. Divination was widely practised in a military context in the Greek world: Pritchett (1979) 47–90; Jameson (1991) 197–228.

For divination in the Roman world Bouché-Leclerq (1879–1882) is still seminal; Pease (1920–1923; repr. 1963) illuminates many cryptic aspects of Cicero's *De Divinatione*, the first known discussion of divination in Roman literature; also useful are Champeaux (1990a) 271ff., 801ff., and Desanti (1990).

> une conséquence naturelle, sinon nécessaire, dès l'on considère cette science comme pouvent contribuer au bonheur de l'homme ou à son perfectionnement moral.[126]

The commonest method was by interpreting the flights of birds,[127] and in Homeric times this task was already vested in the hands of professional augurs,[128] though lay people like Helen,[129] and the Seven Persian conspirators against Smerdis, were also fit for the task.[130]

Μάντις is the usual Greek word for 'seer' or 'prophet' and this is the case all through antiquity since Homeric times.[131] Usually a μάντις is an attribute of a human who communicates the word of god through divine inspiration.[132] By the skill of the seer (μαντικὴ τέχνη) one was likely not only to proclaim divine words but also to have access to divine knowledge. Some Greeks associated μάντις with μαίνεσθαι which means being insane and therefore the notion of prophetic insanity with that of the inspiration of the poet.[133] Plato often speaks of prophecies as manifestations of madness and as resulting from divine inspiration and not from logical reasoning.[134] However, unlike in myth and literature, the μάντιδες in historical times did not actively engage in prophesy. Instead, their realm was primarily the interpretation of signs.[135] Here the key skills are interpreting the entrails of animals, the flights of birds and dreams.

Aristides shared the almost universal belief in the possibility of divination. He appealed to oracles,[136] believed that Asclepius and other deities sent him dreams regarding his health and other matters, and compared the curative powers of the Sacred Well in the precinct of the Pergamene Asclepieion to the prophetic powers of other wells elsewhere.[137] Aristides

---

[126] Bouché-Leclercq (1879) 7.
[127] Hom. *Od.* 2.182.
[128] Hom. *Il.* 1.69; 6.76.
[129] Hom. *Od.* 15.160–181.
[130] Hdt. 3.76.
[131] Cf. Hom. *Il.* 1.62; *Od.* 17.384.
[132] Cf. Aesch. *Choeph.* 559.
[133] Cf. Eur. *Bacch.* 299; Pl. *Phdr.* 244c.
[134] Pl. *Apol.* 22a; *Men.* 99; *Tim.* 71e.
[135] Cf. Paus. 1.34.4.
[136] Aristid. *Or.* 49.12, 38 K.
[137] ἀλλὰ καὶ τἆλλα ὁ θεὸς αὐτῷ χρῆται ὥσπερ ἄλλῳ τῳ συνεργῷ, καὶ πολλοῖς ἤδη πολλάκις τὸ φρέαρ τοῦτο συνεβάλετο εἰς τὸ τυχεῖν ὧν ἔχρῃζον παρὰ τοῦ θεοῦ. ὥσπερ γὰρ οἱ παῖδες οἱ τῶν ἰατρῶν τε καὶ τῶν θαυματοποιῶν γεγυμνασμένοι πρὸς τὰς διακονίας εἰσὶ καὶ συμπράττοντες ἐκπλήττουσι τοὺς θεωμένους καὶ χρωμένους, οὕτω τοῦ μεγάλου θαυματοποιοῦ καὶ πάντα ἐπὶ σωτηρίᾳ πράττοντος ἀνθρώπων εὕρημα τοῦτο καὶ κτῆμά ἐστι καὶ συμπράττει δὴ πρὸς ἅπαντα αὐτῷ

also eulogised Zeus,[138] Athena and Apollo for communicating divine knowledge to humans.[139] On a personal level, the *Sacred Tales* relate a long and continuous relationship between Asclepius (and at times other deities) and Aristides, mainly through dreams, but also in the form of visions and oracles. Aristides' understanding of the nature of the gods as essentially good and helpful,[140] alongside their role as guardians and patrons of mankind, is what made the possibility of divination so reasonable to Aristides.[141]

During his *cathedra*, at the height of his illness, Aristides composed his speech *In Defence of Oratory*. It is an interesting attempt to rehabilitate oratory from the critique of the Platonic Socrates, voiced mainly in the *Gorgias* and the *Phaedrus*. The value of the speech does not lie in its attempts to refute Plato—Aristides deviated from the Platonic themes and arguments, most-likely knowingly, at a rather early stage of the work. The speech does, however, capture much of its author's state of mind at this fragile stage of his illness and career, notwithstanding some of his most elaborate comments on knowledge through divination. Aristides pronounces here his explicit preference for medical knowledge which comes through divination to that which physicians can offer. 'Medicine' Aristides proclaimed, 'which has studied all human science and which is greater than cookery, is feeble, I think, in contrast to the cures of Delphi, which privately and publicly have been revealed to men for all diseases and sufferings'.[142]

καὶ γίγνεται πολλοῖς ἀντὶ φαρμάκου. πολλοὶ μὲν γὰρ τούτῳ λουσάμενοι ὀφθαλμοὺς ἐκομίσαντο, πολλοὶ δὲ πιόντες στέρνον ἰάθησαν καὶ τὸ ἀναγκαῖον πνεῦμα ἀπέλαβον, τῶν δὲ πόδας ἐξώρθωσε, τῶν δὲ ἄλλο τι. ἤδη δέ τις πιὼν ἐξ ἀφώνου φωνὴν ἀφῆκεν, ὥσπερ οἱ τῶν ἀπορρήτων ὑδάτων πιόντες μαντικοὶ γιγνόμενοι.

'But the god also uses it [i.e. the Sacred Well] in other ways like any other co-worker, and the Well has often assisted many people in obtaining from the god what they desired. For just as the sons of doctors and magicians have been trained to serve them and while they aid them astound spectators and customers, so this Well is the discovery and possession of the great magician who does everything for the safety of mankind. It aids him in everything and for many men is like a drug. For many by bathing in it have recovered their sight, and many by drinking it have cured chest trouble and have regained the breath of life ... just as those who have drunk the forbidden waters and have become prophetic'. Aristid. *Or.* 39.14–15 K.

[138] Aristid. *Or.* 43.21–23 K.

[139] Apollo and Athena: Aristid. *Or.* 37. 37.22 K; Apollo gives oracles to mankind: Aristid. *Or.* 37. 37.25 K.

[140] Cf. 'He [i.e. Asclepius] has no leisure to do anything other than to save mankind' (καὶ οὔτε ἐκεῖνος ἄγει σχολὴν ἄλλο τι πράσσειν ἢ σῴζειν ἀνθρώπους). Aristid. *Or.*39.11 K.

[141] Like the author of Ps. Plut. *Placita Philosophorum* 5.1 what Aristides understood by divination is a direct path to god, rather than the technical means for obtaining it.

[142] καίτοι μικρὰ μὲν ἡ πάντας εἰδυῖα λόγους ἀνθρωπίνους ἰατρικὴ καὶ κρείττων ὀψοποιικῆς πρὸς τὰς ἐκ Δελφῶν, οἶμαι, δύναται λύσεις, ὅσαι καὶ ἰδίᾳ καὶ κοινῇ καὶ νόσων καὶ παθημάτων ἁπάντων ἀνθρώποις ἐφάνθησαν. Aristid. *Or.* 2.35 L-B.

Aristides' preference for divine knowledge and for divination as a means to obtain it found much support in Greek tradition.[143] According to Aristides, divine knowledge gained by means of prophecy and divination was proven by Greek history to produce the best constitutions and legislation:

> βαδίζουσί γε εἰς Δελφοὺς καὶ πυνθάνονται περὶ τῶν πολιτειῶν. καὶ τότε τοὺς νόμους τίθενται πρὸς τὴν ἐλθοῦσαν παρὰ τῆς Πυθίας φωνὴν ἀπὸ Λυκούργου πρώτου, τὸν μετὰ πολλοὺς εἰ δεῖ πρῶτον εἰπεῖν χάριν τοῦ λόγου. οὔκουν φασί γ' ἐκεῖνον οὐδὲν θεῖναι Λακεδαιμονίοις ἄνευ τῆς παρὰ τοϋ θεοῦ φωνῆς.[144]
>
> Men go to Delphi to inquire about constitutions. And they legislate according to the voice which comes from the Pythian priestess, beginning with Lycurgus, who came after many others, but must be called first for the sake of argument. Therefore they say that man legislated nothing for the Lacedaemonians without the god's voice.

The application of an argument such as this in a work of rhetoric, which called for a brilliant reworking of familiar themes, demonstrates that the appeal of oracles among Aristides' prospective audience was not a thing of the past, even if the examples themselves were taken from classical Greek history.

It is through divination that Aristides gained much of his divine knowledge and knowledge of the divine. However, his experience and mindset were in no way unique. On the contrary, divination was a familiar institution throughout classical antiquity and Aristides' healing experience, according to his own testimony, is similar to that of many others:

> ἀλλ' ὡς ἀληθῶς ὥσπερ οἱ θεομάντεις οἱ τοῖς τῶν πραγμάτων ἐπωνύμοις τετελεσμένοι παρ' αὐτῶν τῶν θεῶν ἔχω τὸ μάθημα, ὑφ' ὧν ἃ μηδεὶς ἰατρῶν μήτε οἶδεν ὅ τι χρὴ προσειπεῖν, οὐχ ὅπως ἰάσασθαι, μήτ' εἶδεν ἐν ἀνθρώπου φύσει συμβάντα, ἄλλοτ' ἄλλαις παραμυθίαις τε καὶ συμβουλαῖς ἐκ τοῦ θεοῦ διαφεύγων ζῶ παρὰ πᾶν τὸ ἐκ τῶν παρόντων εἰκός. πολλοὶ δ' ἔμοιγε καὶ ἄλλοι κοινωνοί τε καὶ μάρτυρές εἰσι τῶν λόγων, οὐ μόνον τῶν Ἑλλήνων, ἀλλὰ καὶ βαρβάρων, αἵ τ' ἐν Ἀσκληπιοῦ τῶν ἀεὶ διατριβόντων ἀγέλαι καὶ ὅσοι τῷ κατ' Αἴγυπτον θεῷ συνεγένοντο.[145]
>
> Truly just as the seers, initiated into the service of the gods who have given their name to their speciality, I have knowledge from the gods themselves.

---

[143] Aristides had many famous precedents from Greek history which might have encouraged him to put his faith in the hands of the gods in this particular fashion. Sophocles *OT* 897–910 considered the challenge of oracles as equivalent to questioning religion itself and Xenophon listed oracles and predictive dreams among the benefactions the gods bestowed upon mankind: Xen. *Symp*. 4.48; *Mem*. 1.4.15–16; 4.3.12; *Cyr*. 8.7.3; *Eq*. 9.8.

[144] Aristid. *Or*. 2.38–39 L-B.

[145] Aristid. *Or*. 2.67–68 B-L.

> Through their aid, contrary to the likelihood of the circumstances, I am alive, having escaped at different times through various kinds of consolation and advice on the part of the god, from things no doctor knew what to call, to say nothing of cure, nor had seen befall the nature of man. There are many others like me and they can bear witness to these tales, not only Greeks, but barbarians, both the flocks of those who dwell at times in the temple of Asclepius and all those who attend upon the god of Egypt.

According to Aristides the seer forms a picture, but he differs from all others who form pictures because 'all men can form a picture, but the seer can make it into a science ... the whole mantic art is the action of forming a picture [i.e. of knowing the future]'.[146]

Dreams

Belief in divination through dreams was widespread throughout classical antiquity. The Greek and the Latin languages even had words specifically relating to this activity and nouns describing its practitioners.[147] Religiously guided professionals who interpreted dreams had already appeared by the fifth century BCE,[148] and at the same period we find the first of many treatises on the interpretation of dreams.[149] These works discussed the dream-mechanism, collected recurrent dream-patterns, suggested interpretations and instructed those who engaged in the interpretation of dreams how to achieve the best results.[150] The belief in the power of divination through dreams in classical antiquity was encouraged by the prevailing notions about the dream-phenomenon itself. As has already been mentioned, it

---

146 Aristid. *Or.* 2.163–166 B-L.

147 ὀνειροκρισία is the interpretation of dreams and ὀνειροκρίτης is the practitioner. The equivalent Latin terms are: *coniectura, interpretatio*, for dream interpreter and *coniector, interpres* for the person practising.

148 Ar. *Vesp.* 52; Theoph. *Char.* 16.

149 Epicharmus (*apud* Tert. *De. An.* 46); Panyassis of Halicarnassus (*apud* Artem. 1.2.64); Antiphon (*apud* Cic. *De Div.* 1.20.51); Senec. *Controv.* 9; Diog. Laert. 2.46; Lucian, *Hist. Ver.* 2; Tert. *De An.* 46; Hermogen. *De Ideis.* 2.7; Straton (*apud* Diog. Laert. 5.59; Tert. *De An.* 46); Demetrius of Phaleron (*apud* Artem. 2.44); Aristander of Telmessus (*apud* Plin. *Nat. Hist.* 17.38, 343; Plut. *Alex.* 2; Arrian, *Anab.* 2.18; Lucian, Philops. 21–22; Artemid. 1.31, 4.23); Apollodorus of Telmessus (*apud* Artemid. 1.79); Philochorus (*apud* Tert. *De An.* 46); Chrysippus (*apud* Cic. *De Div.* 1.3, 20, 2.65, 70); Antipater of Tarsus (*apud* Cic. *De Div.* 2.70; Artemid. 4.65); Dionysius of Rhodes (*apud* Tert. *De An.* 46; Artemid. 2.66); Cratippus (*apud* Tert. *De An.* 46); Alexander of Myndus (Artemid. 1.67, 2.9, 66); P. Nigidius Figulus (*apud* Io. Lyd. *De Ostent.* 45); Hermippus of Berytus (*apud* Tert. *De An.* 46); Artemon of Miletus (*apud* Artemid. 4.23); Horus (*apud* D.Chr. *Or.* 11) Dio Cassius 72.23.

150 Unfortunately, though, all ancient works on the interpretation of dreams are now lost except that of Artemidorus.

was common in the Graeco-Roman world to perceive the dream-experience as existing objectively in space, and independently of the dreamer.[151] This belief about the nature of dreams explains the popularity of 'oracle dreams' which prevailed all through classical antiquity.[152]

Philosophy is also, to some extent, responsible for the spread of a belief in the predictive nature of dreams and of their medical usage.[153] Plutarch, for example, referred to dreams as the 'oldest oracles'.[154] The Stoic and Pythagorean schools both advocated a rational basis for the significance of dreams. Dreams were particularly relevant in Stoic philosophy. The Stoics associated dreams with their notion of *sympátheia*, which played a vital role in the Stoic philosophical system.[155] The Roman biographer Suetonius, who was generally well-disposed towards the use of dreams to foretell the future,[156] informs us of how the Pythagorean philosopher, Nigidius Figulus, prophesied through dreams the future glory of Augustus' reign.[157] Cicero, in his dialogue *De Divinatione*, which is our most elaborate discussion of the comprehension and use of dreams in the Graeco-Roman world up to his day, also provides firm evidence for the widespread belief in the divine nature of dreams.[158] The book has Cicero and his brother Quintus arguing for and against divination. In the first book Quintus advocates for the validity of divination with an appeal to experience, philosophers, and the general public. The second book presents Marcus arguing against divination through dreams by applying sceptical reason and through showing that no external god or internal soul causes dreams. To Quintus' assertion that dreams may be clairvoyant, precognitive, or veridical,[159] Marcus replies that the outcomes of these dreams are purely fortuitous and are caused by daytime residues and emotions.[160]

---

151 Bouché-Leclercq (1879) 280–290; Dodds (1951) 104; Cox-Miller (1994) 39–78 and see above, 'Dreams'.

152 Harris (2003); Cox Miller (1994).

153 According to Ps. Plut. *Placita Philosophorum* 5.1 Platonists and Stoics perceived divination as a motion towards 'that which is full of the god'. The author said of Epicurus and Xenophanes that they objected the truthfulness of divination. Pythagoras, according to the same author, was dubious as to the practical applications of the *art* of divination, but accepted the possibility of communicating with the gods.

154 Plut. *Sept. Sag.* 15.

155 Cf. Cic. *De Div.* 1.6 discussing Chrysippus and Poseidonius.

156 Wallace-Hadrill (1983) 189–197.

157 Suet. *Aug.* 94. 5.

158 Though the dialogue is set in Rome, between two Roman interlocutors, it rests mainly on Greek works. For recent discussion of this work see: Schofield (1986); Beard (1986).

159 Cic. *De Div.* 1. 58–59.

160 Cic. *De Div.* 2. 140–141.

The view which Marcus presented in the second book of *De Divinatione* did not prevail. Dreams were a major theme for future generations of Graeco-Roman authors,[161] and nowhere was the role of dreams more seminal than in classical historiography. Diodorus Siculus,[162] Dionysius of Halicarnassus,[163] Valerius Maximus,[164] Josephus,[165] Tacitus,[166] Cassius Dio,[167] and Ammianus all introduced them into their works.[168] Suetonius is notable in this respect. He uses dreams to explain the particular course of Roman history and he presents typical attitudes towards dreams of other groups in the Roman world such as Jews, Christians, and Egyptians, as well as Greeks and Romans.[169] In a letter to Suetonius, Pliny recommended that he interpret his own dreams and drew Suetonius' attention to other lawyers who did so.[170] Even the Roman emperor, Marcus Aurelius, accepted a cure given in a dream.[171] His tutor, Fronto, agreed wholeheartedly.[172]

The discussion of dreams and their interpretation in classical antiquity occurred in the context of philosophy, medicine, and religion, mantic and magic. When Aristides related to his dreams as messages from a deity he was not introducing any new ideas about the nature of dreams. In fact, there are even divine patrons of this activity. The interpretation of dreams fell under the jurisdiction of Apollo and Prometheus,[173] and Christine Walde has commented that in both cases 'myth encryptation and the need for interpretation of dream-images served to secure the gods their empowering knowledge. Against this background, dream interpretation by mortals becomes a subversive act of enlightenment'.[174] Viewed more broadly, dreams formed an inherent part of the dialogue between mortals and gods and divination through dreams played a prominent role in Greek theology.

161 Cf. Virgil; Ovid; Propertius, Tibullus, and Seneca. Oberhelman (1993) 146.
162 Diod. Sic. 1. 25. 5; 1. 57. 3–4; 1. 65. 5–8.
163 Dion. Hal. *Ant. Rom.* 1. 53. 3; 1. 57. 3–4; 7. 68. 4.
164 Val. Max. 1. 7.
165 Joseph. *AJ.* 1. 341–342; 11. 326–335; 20. 18–19; *BJ.* 2. 112.
166 Tac. *Ann.* 4. 83; 16. 1–3.
167 Cass. Dio 41. 28; 47. 41; 55. 1. 3–4; 69. 2. 1; 75. 3. 1.
168 Amm. Marc. 15. 3. 5.
169 Oberhelman (1991) chapter 1.
170 Plin. *Ep.* 1. 18.
171 M. Ant. 9. 27.
172 Fronto, *Ep.* 3. 9. 1.
173 Eur. *IT.* 1234–1275; Aesch. *PV.* 476ff.
174 Walde, *DNP* 4, 715.

Dreams dominate the religious experience of Aristides, as well as his healing process. When convalescing in the Pergamene Asclepieion he wrote that in order to obtain cures from the gods it is advisable to use dreams.[175] In the *Sacred Tales* alone Aristides recorded more than 130 such god-sent dreams. Interestingly, Aristides had no difficulty recognising the divine origin of these dreams. In fact, it seemed so self-evident to him that he never cast doubt upon this point. Moreover, the contents of these dreams were accessible to him, either by himself, or through the help of others.

The contents of Asclepius' first dream-revelation to Aristides, c. December, 144 CE, can help us understand the social mechanism which helped him to see the divine authorship of his dreams. In his dream the god ordered Aristides 'to go forth unshod. And I cried in my dream, as if in a waking state and after the accomplishment of the dream: "Great is Asclepius! The order is accomplished."'[176] At the time Aristides was sick and bewildered, having been offered no cure or even prognosis by the physicians in Smyrna, and was convalescing in the warm springs of Pergamum, near the famous Pergamene Asclepieion.[177] The god, who was well known for his dream-therapies and particularly eminent in the vicinity of his renowned and newly renovated temple, was also known for prescribing this exact remedy.[178] Hence it is more than plausible that Aristides was particularly attentive to this kind of a message from Asclepius at this time and in this place. Moreover, the social and cultural environment Aristides inhabited supported his interpretation of dreams as divine messages.[179] Even his physicians, in the Asclepieion and elsewhere, were aware of the possibility of divine medical message through dreams and included Asclepius' prescriptions in their prescribed regimen.

During his period in the Pergamene Asclepieion Aristides wrote that in order to procure cures from the god 'we employ dreams, not knowing in advance of the evening, surely, what we are going to see, and we know

---

175 Aristid. *Or.* 2.70 L-B.

176 ἀνυπόδητόν τε γὰρ προελθεῖν ἐπέταξε καὶ ἐβόων δὴ ἐν τῷ ὀνείρατι ὡς ἂν ὕπαρ τε καὶ ἐπ' ὀνείρατι τετελεσμένῳ, μέγας ὁ 'Ασκληπιός, τετέλεσται τὸ πρόσταγμα. Aristid. *Or.* 48.7 K.

177 As said before (pp. 48–49) providing an accurate prognosis was the best method for a physician to gain his patient's trust. The inability of Aristides' physicians to do that must have diminished his faith in them from the very beginning of his illness and might have led Aristides to the Asclepieion in the first place.

178 Cf. M.Ant. 5.8.1 (Quoted above, p. 119, n. 461).

179 Moreover, if one is to accept Freud's notion of the secondary dream, which I have discussed above, it is likely that the fact that this was Aristides' recollection of the dream is also indicative of the social setting in which he lived.

what we must do to be saved, although we are ignorant up to that minute in which the benefit has come from the god'.[180] Aristides' reassurance that 'we know what we must do to be saved' (σωθῆναι γιγνώσκομεν) must have been supported by the establishment of the temple. The votive offerings in the temple emphasised to those present that the god had helped his worshippers many times before.[181] The practice of incubation encouraged patients to perceive all their dreams during their stay in the Asclepieion as being god-sent. The temple-priests nourished this belief, helped the patients to interpret their dreams as divine messages and authenticated their divine origin.

Oracles

Amongst the various forms of divination practised by the Greeks, the responses of a deity or a hero given in an oracular site were the most prestigious.[182] Greek tradition has it that oracles provided prophecies on a wide range of issues, from politics to personal prospects.[183] Healing oracles also existed, particularly ones associated with Asclepius. However, even in these sites the oracles were not restricted to medical matters and divine help concerning medical issues was not procured solely from the oracles associated with Asclepius. For example, in the *Sacred Tales* Aristides records that during his illness:

> ἐνθύμιον γίγνεταί μοι χρήσασθαι τῷ θεῷ τῷ ἐν Κολοφῶνι καὶ περὶ τῶν παρόντων καὶ περὶ πάσης τῆς ἀσθενείας. ἀπέχει δὲ ἡ Κολοφὼν τῆς Λεβέδου οὐ πολὺ, καὶ ἡ νὺξ ἐτύγχανεν ἡ ἱερὰ ἐπικειμένη. δόξαν ταῦτα, πέμπω τὸν Ζώσιμον. ἐπελθούσης δὲ τῆς νυκτὸς τῷ μὲν Ζωσίμῳ γίγνεται τόδε τὸ μαντεῖον φέρον εἰς ἐμὲ
>
> Ἰήσεταί σε νοῦσον ἠδ' ἀκέσσεται
>
> Ἀσκληπιὸς, πόλισμα Τηλέφου κλυτὸν
>
> τιμῶν, Καίκου ναμάτων οὐ τηλόθεν.[184]

---

180 ἀλλὰ καὶ ὀνείρασι χρώμεθα οὐ προειδότες, οἶμαι, τῆς ἑσπέρας ὅ τι μέλλομεν ὄψεσθαι, καὶ τί χρὴ ποιήσαντας σωθῆναι γιγνώσκομεν ἀγνοοῦντες μέχρι ἐκείνου τοῦ μέρους τῆς ὥρας, ἐν ᾧ παρὰ τῶν θεῶν ἧκε τἀγαθὸν. Aristid. *Or.* 2.70 L-B.

181 Renberg (2003) *passim*; Petsalis-Diomidis (2005) 213 ff.

182 Cf. Soph. *OT*. 498–501.

183 Individuals enquire, for example, if their wife will conceive (and whether it will be a boy or a girl), if a proposed journey, career change or marriage is wise, whether a child is legitimate; they also enquired about health problems and, in a more general tone, how to keep the favour of the gods. The reply would have been either a 'yes', a 'no' or 'by sacrificing x'. *OCD*[3] s.v. Oracles; Price (1999) 73–76; Parke (1967); Parke (1985); Price (2004); Parker (1983) and (1996).

184 Aristid. *Or.* 49.12 K.

> It occurred to me to consult the god in Colophon [i.e. the oracle][185] both concerning my present troubles [i.e. legal issues] and general weakness. Colophon is not far from Lebedus, and the Sacred Night happened to be near. Since it seemed to me best to do this, I sent Zosimus. When the night came, Zosimus received the following oracle, which pertained to me: "Asclepius will cure and heal your disease/in honour of the famous city of Telephus/not far from the streams of the Caicus".

Aristides records consultation of oracles about public issues as well. For example, after September, 149 CE, there were frequent earthquakes in Asia and the Ephesians and the Smyrnaeans sent emissaries to the oracle of Apollo at Clarus.[186]

Although these are the only two records we know of that concern consultations with an oracle from Aristides' own lifetime (only one of which related directly to him), he was familiar with a wide range of famous oracular pronouncements from Greek history.[187] Moreover, Aristides did not seem to have drawn any distinction between the origin and validity of oracular pronouncements and that of god-sent dreams.[188] He opens his *Sacred Tales* with this statement of purpose: 'to record the events or narrate the providence of the god, wherein he revealed some things openly in his own presence, others by sending dreams'.[189] It is a personal narrative of divination. However, the *Sacred Tales* did not strike its ancient readership as eccentric or odd.[190] Divine interventions in the lives of mankind were not uncommon in classical antiquity. The manner in which Aristides communicated with the gods was far from innovative. On the contrary, his descriptions of divination follow traditional models, much like his appeals to oracles and to the healing cult of Asclepius. Aristides' experience of divination, like his religious experience as a whole, was shaped by society. Aristides did not have to coin a term for divination. It was in society that he learned how to invoke the gods through incubation and appeal to oracles; it was priests and his cultural heritage which guided him in the process of identifying divine messages in his dreams and visions; it was society which offered Aristides the tools to interpret these messages. Divination was probably a private experience in a psychological sense, but all his conceptualisation and understanding of div-

185 The god of Colophon is Apollo of Clarus. Cf. Robert (1969) 305–312.
186 Aristid. *Or.* 49.38 K.
187 Cf. Aristid. *Or.* 1.30, 37, 46, 87, 167, 173, 399, 401 B-L.
188 Aristid. *Or.* 50.75 K.
189 ἀπογράφειν ἐβούλετο, ἢ τὴν τοῦ θεοῦ πρόνοιαν διηγεῖσθαι, ὧν τὰ μὲν ἐκ τοῦ φανεροῦ παρὼν, τὰ δὲ τῇ πομπῇ τῶν ἐνυπνίων ἐνεδείκνυτο. Aristid. *Or.* 47.3 K.
190 See above, 'The Ancient readers of the *Sacred Tales*'.

ination was guided by public institutions. Divination could be someone's private experience only because it had a public meaning and a consensual method of decoding.

The section has focused on the religious experience of Aelius Aristides as this experience is portrayed in the *Sacred Tales*. The point of origin was an alleged cleavage which Graeco-Roman society saw between private or personal religions and public ones. Having considered the conceptual, theological and behavioural components of the religious experience of Aristides, it became evident that the origin of each of these components was external to Aristides. Moreover, they were all taken from the mainstream of Graeco-Roman culture. Aristides' idea of theology, cosmology and cosmogony, as well as his comprehension of the myth of Asclepius itself, were in accordance with the teachings of Graeco-Roman traditions. Even cultic habits, such as the practice of divination and interpretation of dreams, were taught to Aristides by some of the most popular, well-established and distinguished religious centres and institutions of his day (e.g. the priests and attendants in the temples of Asclepius). Furthermore, Aristides' understanding of the way dreams come into being and operate as means of divination received important reinforcement from corroborative disciplines, such as philosophy and medicine. The next section will focus on the *modus operandi* of some of the major agents of Graeco-Roman culture which were responsible for communicating religious themes in Aristides' world and which guaranteed, to a large extent, a common understanding of the divine.

4. Visual Culture and Social Forms of Cult-Organisation

The previous section was dedicated the conceptual scheme which regulated the religious experience of Aelius Aristides and its genealogy in Graeco-Roman thought. In this section I will concentrate on some of the prominent agents which were responsible for transmitting these religious themes in Aristides' world in an attempt both to evaluate their effect on his religious experience and to contextualise it. Wishing to escape the limitations which are posed by relying exclusively on literary sources (these limitations result both from the paucity of relevant literary evidence and the difficulty of employing them to depict a reliable picture of the religious climate during the high empire), this section will focus upon the effects of visual culture and of social forms of cult-organisation on shaping religious experience in Aristides' world.

Cult, Festivals and Games

The forces which influenced the religious experience of Aristides included sets of abstract ideas, such as theology and philosophy, but they also included the social agents of religion in the Graeco-Roman world—cult, festivals and games—which transmitted, regulated and inculcated religious doctrines. Aristides was an enthusiastic participant in religious cult, festivals and feasts, particularly ones dedicated to Asclepius. In his *Sacred Tales* he recorded many occasions on which he himself participated in such events. Moreover, a number of his hymns and epideictic speeches were delivered during festivals and feasts.[191] Many of his other works include some discernable religious themes. In the following section I look into the particular ways in which these religious and social institutions imbued Aristides with religious doctrines.

There is much reverential homage rendered to a divine being in Aristides' work. He seemed to have shared Libanius' view that though the gods are prone to beneficence of their own free will, they are still more inclined to it when invoked.[192] Ancient Graeco-Roman religion is inconceivable without rituals.[193] Cult was perceived as a necessary actualisation of belief.[194] This is particularly true with respect to Asclepius, the god of medicine, whom his worshippers approached when seeking cure. Indeed, Aristides' record of cultic activity in the Asclepieion is not fundamentally different to other testimonies that we have, although it appears that his picture is at times incomplete. Aristides did not, for example, say anything about initiation rites for the cult of Asclepius.[195] He does, however tell us many other things about life in the Asclepieion and the cult which was practised there. To begin with he describes how the running of the temple was entrusted to temple priests

---

191 E.g. Aristid. *Or.* 17 K was delivered at a celebration of the Dionysia in Smyrna; *Or.* 34 K was delivered in the council Chamber of Smyrna during the games of the provincial assembly (as described in *Or.* 51.38–41 K); *Or.* 38 K was delivered in the Pergamene Asclepieion; *Or.* 46 K was delivered in the summer of 166 CE in Corinth, during the Isthmian Games; *Or.* 42 K was delivered in the temple of Zeus-Asclepius in Pergamum, at the celebration of the Night Festival on January 6, 177 CE; *Or.* 45 K was delivered in Smyrna at 142 CE, probably at the festival of Zeus Sarapis.

192 Lib. *Or.* 34.23–26.

193 Edelstein & Edelstein vol. ii (1945) 181.

194 Perhaps the best example of the inherent aspect of ritual in Graeco-Roman religion is the demand that Christians take part in sacrifices to the Emperor. Seen from a 'pagan' point of view, this act was a necessary proof of intentions.

195 There is evidence to support the existence of initiation rites. *IG* IV^2 1, 121; Paus. 5.13.3; *I. Perg.* II 264; Ar. *Plut.* 660–661; *IG* II^2 4962; *IG* IV^2 1, 128; Philostr. *VA* 1.10.

(two during Aristides' convalescence).[196] The priests had jurisdiction over all the servants of the god and those who had posts in the temple, as well as providing medical care for the patients.[197] They were also an authority on dream interpretation.[198] Sacrifices and thank-offerings were also common.[199] Aristides himself dreamt that he sent Asclepius a wreath and candles on two different occasions.[200] Both these votive offerings were common amongst Asclepius' worshippers. Other aspects of the cult, such as cleansing and sacrifices, speeches and feasts, are frequently mentioned in his testimonies and are easily corroborated by other sources. During Aristides' *cathedra* he witnessed the temple priests in their daily routines,[201] such as their lighting of the sacred candles.[202] He also records a dream, probably based on his real experiences, in which: 'I stood at the propylaea of the temple. Many others were also gathered together, as whenever there is a purificatory ceremony at the temple'.[203] These details resemble other descriptions, both

---

[196] Aristid. *Or.* 48.29 K. Temple priests are mentioned already in Ar. *Plut.* 676–681.

[197] Aristid. *Or.* 48.47 K.

[198] Cf. Aristid. *Or.* 48.35 K; Cic. *De Div.* 2.59.

[199] Sacrifices: Aristid. *Or.* 50.6 K; *IG* IV^2, 1, 126. Thank-offerings: Ael. *Fr.* 101; Callim. *Epigr.* 55. An inscription from Erythrae describes a law concerning cult of Asclepius and Apollo, with hymns to Apollo and Asclepius in verse, stoichedon; 380/360 BC (but ll. 74–76 c. 281 BC); found there (copies of hymn to Asclepius also found at Athens and at Ptolemais in Egypt): *ADAW* 1909, pp. 37–48, no. 11; *SEG* 4, 626; Sokolowski, *LSAM* 24; *SEG* 15, 719; *I.Ery* 205; see also the discussion in Furley and Bremer vol. i. (2001) 212 ff. This paean has also been found at three other locations; in all three the inscriptions are dated to the Roman era: i. an Egyptian inscription from Ptolemais Herion in the Thebaid can be dated to 97 AD; ii. An Athenian inscription (*IG* III 1, 171) which can be dated to the 1st or 2nd century AD; iii. An inscription from Dion in Macedonia that can be dated to the 2nd century CE (editions and studies are discussed in Furley and Bremer vol. ii. (2001) 161 ff.). Inscriptions from the Pergamene Asclepieion record many examples of thank offerings cf. Habicht (1969) nos. 67, 68, 73, 74 which were dedicated by Roman magistrates in Latin. No. 69 is a thank offering to Asclepius for his prescription of remedy. Payment of vows to Asclepius, presumably after successful treatments were also common, cf. nos. 70, 82, 83, 86, 87, 90, 99, 108, 110, 111a, 111b, 111c, 115b. No. 71 is a thank offering to Asclepius and Hygieia for protecting one Attalus, son of the Pergamene Attalus from many perils. No. 72 is a thank offering of a lady, following a divine behest. This inscription also includes a catalogue of votive offerings, such as five bronze and four silver human figures (lines 7 ff., with Habicht ad loc.). Some thank offerings were explicitly made following a dream, cf. nos. 75, 76, 91, 116, 117. No. 79 is a thank offering of a consul, who was also a worshipper of Asclepius.

[200] Wreath: Aristid. *Or.* 47.44 K; candles: Aristid. *Or.* 47.32 K.

[201] Aristid. *Or.* 47.11; 48.29 K.

[202] Aristid. *Or.* 47.11 K.

[203] ἐδόκουν ἐν τοῖς προπυλαίοις ἑστάναι τοῦ ἱεροῦ, συνειλέχθαι δὲ καὶ ἄλλους πολλούς τινας, ὥσπερ ἡνίκα ἂν τὸ ἱερὸν καθάρσιον γίγνηται. Aristid. *Or.* 48.31 K.

written contemporaneously and earlier.[204] The priests at the Asclepieion of Cos, for example, are mentioned by the third century BCE Hellenistic poet Herodas.[205] The white garment Aristides mentioned is also referred to by Isyllus, the third century BCE poet from Epidaurus.[206] It appears, then, that the habits Aristides recorded were in no way unique or novel.

Most Asclepieia shared common features, which reflected a common understanding of the myth. The children of Asclepius, his sons Machaon and Podalirius, and his daughter Hygieia, featured in the cult in most Asclepieia, as did Apollo, whose name appears in the official inscriptions from Epidaurus and always came before that of Asclepius. A central feature of the cult was incubation,[207] which was practised in the expectation of receiving dreams in which the god prescribed healing.[208] Often actual therapy followed and the Asclepieia developed into what can be referred to as hospitals.[209]

It is also noteworthy that members of the medical staff connected with the Pergamene Asclepieion were also responsible for the development of sophistic studies. Pergamum was the home of several important sophists. One of them, Aristocles, was a Roman consul who returned to Pergamum to further his studies and remained in the city to teach.[210] Glen Bowersock has argued that the city's appeal for sophists had much to do with the medical staff of the Asclepieion.[211] Pergamum was no exception. According

---

204 The evidence is collected by Edelstain & Edelstein vol. 1 (1945) T 484–542.

205 Herod. 4.58.

206 Aristid. *Or.* 48.31 K; *IG* IV^2 1, 128.

207 Iamblichus said that in the Asclepieion illnesses are healed by divine dreams. Through the ordinances of visions that occur at night the medical art was composed from divinely inspired dreams. Iambl. *Myst.* Philostratus' Apollonius made his way to Pergamum in order to teach how to obtain favourable dreams (Philostr. *VA* 4.11). Even Cicero took this habit for granted, even if his persona in the *De Div.* was critical about it (Cic. *De Div.* 2.59). Needless to say, Aristides was deeply devout (*Or.* 47.57, 48.31–35 K). To this literary evidence we must add the considerable number of inscriptions. For collections of relevant evidence see Deubner (1900) who was mainly interested in the practice of incubation and its adaptation by Christians; Edelstein and Edelstein vol. i (1945) who focused on the cult of Asclepius, as did Graf (1992) 186–193; for Pergamum see Wörrle (1969) no. 161; the healing inscriptions were discussed by Guarducci (1978) 143–166, with the addition of Müller (1987) 193–233. Renberg (2003) looked into votive offerings, dedicated after a vision of a deity took place.

208 Cf. Ar. *Plut.* 400–414, 633–747; Ael. *NA.* 9.33; *IG* IV^2 1, 121–122; *IG* IV^2 1, 127; Oribasius, *Collectiones Medicae*, 45.30.10–14; *I. Cret.* 1.17. no. 9.

209 The term was not used by contemporaries. In fact, excluding the Roman military *valetudinaria*, there were no hospitals until the Byzantine era.

210 He was important enough for Philostratus to include him in his collection of sophists' biographies: Philostr. *VS* 567–568. See further Halfmann (1979).

211 Bowersock (1969) 19, 66–67.

to Philostratus, Apollonius, the philosopher-sage from Tyana, migrated to the temple of Asclepius in the town of Aegeae 'where Asclepius reveals himself in person to men' (καὶ ὁ 'Ασκληπιακὸς αὐτος ἐπίδηλος τοῖς ἀνθρώποις) to benefit from the philosophical teaching there.[212] The priests in Pergamum were descendants of the Asclepiads, their position was a lifetime office and they were in charge of liturgy, supervision of the buildings, and financial accounts.[213] By the time of Aristides, this office was held by the family of C. Julius Apellas whose sons were the priests of Asclepius.[214] During his *cathedra* Aristides resided with Asclepiacus, one of the temple's wardens, in his house, which lay outside the precinct.[215]

The consideration of cultic habits in a work which studies Aristides' religious experience hardly needs justification. The work of sociologists shows how particular patterns of cult which were moulded over time by society dictate both the form as well as the content of its participants' religious experience.[216] At the time Aristides was resident, services were held in the temple twice a day, at which Sacred Lamps were lit. Before arriving at the temple for incubation or prayer the worshipper performed a ritual washing for purification.[217] Ritual washings with water from the Sacred Well and wearing white clothes were part of the regular rites of the temple.[218] Prayers and choral hymns accompanied by a cithara were central aspects of its liturgy.[219] Speeches were also composed and delivered at the Sacred Theatre.[220] Sacrifices, vows and votive offerings, which represented parts of the bodies of the diseased, were also common.[221]

At stated periods, probably in January and August, great festivals were held in Pergamum, with games, poetic contests, and nightly vigils held in honour of the god.[222] Festivals in honour of Asclepius dated back to the fifth

---

212 Philostr. *VA* 1.7.

213 *I. Perg.* II 251; Aristid. *Or.* 30. 13–15, 25, 27 K.

214 Behr (1968) 30–31, and Habicht (1969) no. 45.

215 Aristid. *Or.* 48. 35, 46 K. For the epigraphical evidence concerning the temple priests see Habicht (1969) nos. 45–55.

216 Particularly illuminating in this respect are the works of Geertz, such as 'Thick description: Toward an Interpretative Theory of Culture' and 'Religion as a Cultural System', both in Geertz (1973).

217 Aristid. *Or.* 51. 28 K; Paus. 5.13.3; *I. Perg.* II 264.

218 Aristid. *Or.* 39. 17 K; 48. 31; *IG* IV^2 1 128.

219 Aristid. *Or.* 48. 7; 50. 50 K.

220 Such an oration is Aristid. *Or.* 42 K.

221 Aristid. *Or.* 47. 44, 45 K; Liv. 40. 37; *I. Perg.* II 264; *IMT* 4.

222 Behr (1968) 32 n. 47.

century BCE.[223] For the Greeks, one way of dealing with the multiplicity of their gods was a firm structure of various calendars of festivals and sacrifices.[224] Sacrifices were always accompanied by prayers, which explained the purpose of the sacrifice and named what was requested from the deity in return.[225] In addition to sacrifices, hymns were often sung during the festivals. The standard structure was invocation of the gods, honouring them by narrating some of their divine deeds, and finally praying for their godly favour.[226] It was common all through the Hellenistic and Roman periods to have special choirs to sing hymns to the gods. Aristides himself composed such hymns and conducted a choir of boys who sang them.[227] He also records hymns composed by others,[228] and that others conducted hymns he himself composed.[229] Two other mentions of his hymns are made in the *Sacred Tales*,[230] and many other hymns to Asclepius have also been recorded.[231] Cult hymns deployed, of course, mythological themes and were considered to be an inherent part of the cult. Many of these hymns were recorded on stone and an exceptionally worthy hymn was considered in itself a gift to the god.[232] In Roman times, in addition to lyric hymns, the orators also composed prose ones. Aristides himself composed ten such prose hymns to the gods, and books guiding orators wishing to perform such a task were at hand.[233]

Festivals were a centre of communication and one of the most important public occasions in the Greek world, transforming a group of people

---

223 Epidaurus: Pind. *Nem.* 5.95–97; *Scholia in Pindarum, Nem.* 3.147, 5.94b, 96; Pl. *Ion*, 530a; *IG* IV² 1. 40, 41, 47. Athens: Paus. 2.26.8; Philostr. *VA* 4.18; Aeschin. 3.66–67; Arist. *Ath. Pol.*, 56.4. Cos: Hippoc. *Ep.* 11. Pergamum: Lucian, *Icar.* 24; Aristid. *Or.* 47.6, 48.74 K. Lampsacus, *IMT* 4. Ephesus: *I. Eph.* 1162. Italy: Arn. *Adv. Nat.* 7.32; Pollux, *Onomasticon*, 1.37.

224 Price (1999) 25.

225 Price (1999) 34.

226 Price (1999) 37.

227 Aristid. *Or.* 49.4 K.

228 Aristid. *Or.* 48.21 K.

229 Aristid. *Or.* 50.42 K.

230 Aristid. *Or.* 50.44, 47.73 K.

231 *IG* II² 4510 (Imperial); Lucian, *Dem. Enc.* 27; Philostr. *VA* 3.17; Philostr. *Imag.* 13; *Etymologicum Magnum*, s.v. Δεξίων Anonymus, *Paean Erthyreaeus in Asclepium* (c. 380–360 BC), *IG* II² 4473; *IG* IV² 1 128; Gal. 14.42 K; *IG* 14, 967a, 967b; *Orphei Hymni*, 67; Ath. 6.55.250c; Paus. 3.26.10. On paeans as a literary genre see Rutherford (2001) 3–136; Furley and Bremer (2001). Bowie (2006) adds much to our understanding of the place of paeans in choral performances during the imperial period.

232 Theoc. 22.223; Price (1984) 88; Price (1999) 37.

233 Aristid. *Or.* 47.73; 50.52, 52 K; Price (1999) 46; Quintilian 3.7.7–8; Alexander Numenius, in Spengel, *Rhetores Graeci* 3.4–6; and in the third century Menander Rhetor, 333–344.15 eds. Russell and Wilson.

into a community.[234] They played a vital role in creating a group identity and because most festivals had a religious aspect these events also functioned as guardians of religious tradition. Attendance at festivals and feasts had, therefore, a formative and educative function. Although the study of Greek festivals has for long concentrated on issues of agrarian magic and fertility, no doubt due to the powerful influence of Mannhardt and Frazer, and later Nilsson and Deubner, the social and political aspects of festivals must not be overlooked.[235] Moreover, having been celebrated regularly and collectively they formed a powerful instrument of religious tradition. Asclepius' festivals, which included rites of purification, dedications to the god and invocations for his help, as well as speeches, hymns, the dressing of statues and other customs which associated the god with his myth, conveyed one religious narrative to all participants.

Greek festivals had four distinct sections: firstly, a procession (which often included masked parades); secondly, sacrifices and banquets; thirdly, a choir singing and/or dancing; and finally competitions (ἀγῶνες). Myths attempted to bind rituals together using narrative. However, these narratives always allowed room for change and innovation. Feasts in particular became 'the communicative *locus* in which religion confronted society in nomothetic terms and the poet took on the function of the theologian'.[236] The hymns of Aristides were both part of the educational mechanism of Greek festivals as well as a result of it. Functioning as the *loci* of identity of social groups, festivals and feasts had a leading role in articulating this identity and explaining it in religious terms.

The formative nature of cult, festivals and games is another indicator of the false dichotomy between private and public religions.[237] The influence of socially-organised religion is clearly attested in Aristides' narration of his own illness (an illness which, in itself, was, to a large extent, understood by Aristides in religious terms). His use of medical vocabulary, as well as the fact that some of the prescriptions Asclepius gave Aristides were very common amongst the god's worshippers, demonstrates the influence

234 Auffarth, 'Festivals', *DNP* 5, 399.

235 Frazer (1900); Mannhardt (1904); Nilsson (1906); Deubner (1932). For more recent approaches see Auffarth, 'Festivals', *DNP* 5, 401; Price (1999) 11–46.

236 Auffarth, 'Festivals', *DNP* 5, 401.

237 While it is true that Aelius Aristides presented himself as an exceptional worshipper, the very arguments he used to prove it, his choice to present these arguments in hymns and orations prove the opposite, i.e. that his notions of the god and of proper cultic activities were taught to him by the social institutions in which he was embedded.

of contemporary religious discourse on Aristides' religious experience.[238] The simplest explanation for this influence was that the medical activity in the Asclepieion and the prominent part played by the temple staff (who, notably, were also Asclepius' priests) forced Aristides' most private experiences, namely his reactions to his pathologies and the contents of his dreams, into a general pattern. Furthermore, the dual role of the temple staff as health-care providers and as organisers of religious cult blurred all distinction between the medical and the religious jurisdiction. This socially-organised cult taught an individual worshipper, like Aristides, how to relate to his illness; what he should expect from Asclepius; how to invoke the god; which vocabulary to use in the process; and how to recognise the hand of god when it finally touched his worshipper. The fact that it was not uncommon for Asclepius to prescribe more than one patient the same treatment (in fact, horseback riding and running without shoes were very common) is indicative of the efficiency of the formative role of cult in the Asclepieion.[239] Cult, festivals, and games moulded Aristides' religious experience of being ill into its particular form.

The Power of Images

Aristides' knowledge of theology, his mental image of the gods, and his comprehension of the means of invoking a deity, were shaped not only by reading and listening, but also by seeing. In the last three decades, scholarship within the field of the history of classical art has produced many important contributions to our understanding of how Graeco-Roman art functioned as a mode of communication.[240] For example, Tonio Hölscher

---

[238] See above, chapter 2, section 2.

[239] These forms of cult included various modes of narrating past acts of grace of Asclepius during festivals in various ways; for example, inscribing such narratives as votive-offerings on the temples' stone surface.

[240] Seminal: Hölscher (2004). Hölscher's project is to explore the language of imagery in Roman art as a semantic system. He follows the works of philosophers of language, notably Wittgenstein, in looking for (and actually finding) a grammar for this language. Hölscher described this language as natural language (unlike a formal language). Visual language was not, Hölscher shows, consciously devised. Rather, it evolved gradually and organically, which explains natural inconsistencies in its expression. (p. 2). Zanker (1988) looked into the power of images in the age of Augustus and the ability of images to convey a wide range of delicate messages; Elsner (1991) analyses the Augustan *Ara Pacis* as a part of Augustus' propaganda-efforts, (1992) looks into Pausanias' work as a visual revocation of Greece, (1996) studies the connection between images and ritual in classical antiquity, (2007) examines whether the ancient art of physiognomics influenced the visual arts and vice versa.

has commented that 'the common visual language of society—underlying the thematics of its imagery and regardless of minor temporal and local stylistic differences—is a social fact of the greatest interest'.[241] In his work on *The Language of Images in Roman Art* he has examined how visual works were intended to act as semantic vehicles of communication. Paul Zanker has looked into the visual language or the visual imagery in classical art, which he understands to include not only works of art, buildings and literary imagery, but also religious rituals, clothing, state and regional ceremonies, the emperor's conduct and forms of social intercourse, insofar as they created a visual impression. Zanker is concerned both with the context of these images and with the effect of this assemblage of images upon the viewer. The authors of these studies, though not neglecting the role of production and distribution of works of art in creating a visual language, have paid particular attention to the form—by which they mean both the style and the semantic system (i.e. the elements and their use)[242]—that enabled classical artists to produce visual paradigms, without which art cannot function as means of communication. In this second part of the section I will look into the influence of visual culture on the religious experience of Aristides and will try to identify its imprint on his mental image of the divine and on his cultic habits.

An inquiry into the role of works of visual art as a means of communication and as a form of language is essential to a study of Aristides' religious experience because most Greek art was (to varying degrees) religious in function,[243] and because of the widespread presence of works of art across the Graeco-Roman world.[244] Furthermore, because every aspect of the visual communication that shaped Aristides' religious experience was also a part of this language of images it must have transmitted similar messages to most, if not all, of its viewers. These images therefore provide a much firmer context in which to place the religious experience of Aristides than written works alone can offer. Images such as the marble statue of Asclepius from the Pergamene Asclepieion and a marble votive relief depicting a family of worshippers approaching Asclepius with an offering provided the viewer with a tangible notion of the god, taught viewers how to approach the deity,

241 Hölscher (2004) 1.
242 Hölscher (2004) 58–85.
243 Elsner (1996) 515.
244 Cf. D.Chr. *Or.* 31. In this oration Dio urges the Rhodians to quit their habit of rededicating old statues to new benefactors. It appears from the speech that in the city of Rhodes alone there were more than 3,000 statues and works of art for public display.

and what to expect.[245] The formative effect of works of visual art on Aristides and their function as a mechanism of education and indoctrination can be corroborated by the comments of some of Aristides' contemporary Greek authors. Indeed, Second Sophistic authors produced remarkable aesthetic images[246] and they recorded in their work the impact of art on the Graeco-Roman imagination,[247] especially in respect to ritual, prophecy and magic.[248] Particularly interesting here is the example of Artemidorus, who sees the appearance of a god's statue in a dream as equivalent to the appearance of the god himself. According to Artemidorus, statues of the gods seen in dreams were no different, from the point of view of the dream interpreter, to the gods themselves.[249] Moreover, it was important to be aware of the precise materials from which the divine statue was made[250] and of its position and context[251] if one was to find the correct interpretation of a dream. In effect, in order to predict the future, the dreamer had to develop an acute and precise *visual memory*, sensitive to the aesthetics and attributes of divine statues and cult images.[252]

The ancients ascribed godly powers to images. Referring to a statue of Asclepius, Callistratus, the late antique author of the 'descriptions', wrote:

> Εἶτα τὸ μὲν Ἀργῷον σκάφος ἔμφωνον γενέσθαι πειθόμεθα τὸ ὑπὸ τῶν Ἀθηνᾶς τεχνηθὲν χειρῶν, ὃ καὶ τὴν ἐν ἄστροις ἐκληρούχησε τύχην, ἄγαλμα δὲ οὐ πιστεύσομεν, εἰς ὃ τὰς δυνάμεις Ἀσκληπιὸς ἀνίησι τὸν προνοητικὸν ἐπεισάγων νοῦν ἐπὶ τὴν ἑαυτοῦ κοινωνίαν, τοῦ συνοικοῦντος τὴν δύναμιν πρέπειν, ἀλλ' εἰς μὲν ἀνθρώπινα κατάγεσθαι τὸ θεῖον δώσομεν, ἔνθα καὶ μιανθῆναι παθήμασιν, οὐ πιστεύσομεν δέ, ᾗ μηδὲν ἔγγονον κακίας παραπέφυκεν.[253]

> Are we to believe that the vessel Argo, which was wrought by the hands of Athena and later assumed its allotted place among the stars, became capable of speech, and yet in the case of a statue into which Asclepius infused his

245 Petsalis-Diomidis (2010) figs. 4, 5, with discussion.

246 Elsner (1996) 515; Elsner (2007) 206.

247 Moreover, as we learn from Dio's *Rhodian Oration*, Second Sophistic authors were not unaware of the role of works of visual art as guardians of the past and the potential of manipulating collective memory by changing certain aspects in these works of art (*c.f.* Dio's warning that re-dedication of old statues, which have been dedicated before, will obliterate important chapters of Rhodian history and will, in consequence, alter the Rhodians' perception of who they are).

248 Elsner (1996) 515–516.

249 Artem. 2.35, 39; cf. Barasch, (1992) 32–33.

250 Artem. 2.39.

251 Artem. 2.37.

252 Elsner (1996) 516.

253 Callistratus, *Descriptiones*, 10.1.

> own powers, introducing purposeful intelligence therein and thus making it a partner with himself, not believe that the power of indwelling god is clearly manifest therein? Nay, more, shall we admit that the divine spirit descends into human bodies, there to be even defiled by passions, and nevertheless not to believe it in a case where there is no attendant engendering of evil?

It appears that not only was the visual representation of Asclepius well known in antiquity through the god's many statues, but that actually attributing divine powers to these statues was not uncommon amongst his worshippers.

Images of Asclepius were held in high esteem in classical antiquity. Statues from Epidaurus, Piraeus, Argos, and Cos, as well as coins from Epidaurus, Cos, and Pergamon are but a few examples for the wide presence of the image of Asclepius in art.[254] Pausanias, for example, describing the Asclepieion in Athens, advises his reader to see the statues of the god and his children in the temple.[255] The ancient commentators on statues of Asclepius, much like Aristides himself, were conscious not only of the shape and posture of the statues of Asclepius,[256] but also of the materials from which they were made. Stone, ivory, bronze and gold were the most common materials used.[257] Of Asclepius' image at Aegina, Pausanias says that he is seated,[258] and he described how the image in Epidaurus was made of ivory and gold, and was seated as well.[259] The statue of Asclepius in Epidaurus was included by the anonymous author of *De Incredibilibus* as one of the world's wonders.[260] Of Messene, Pausanias says that 'the most numerous statues and the most worth seeing are to be found in the sanctuary of Asclepius'.[261] The image of Asclepius was also known in Rome where a statue of Asclepius was dedicated by Augustus himself in honour of his

---

254 Statues: Petsalis-Diomidis (2010) figs. 4, 5, 6, 7, 8, 9,10, 15, 16, 17, 18, 1920, 21, 22, and *LIMC*. Kerenyi.

255 Paus. 1.21.4.

256 Posture: upright Paus. 8.32.5 (In Megalopolis); seated: Paus. 2.27.2 (In Epidaurus).

257 At Leuctra: Puas. 3.26.4. At Partae, Achaia: Paus. 7.20.9. At Corinth it was marble: Paus. 2.4.5, like in Phocis: Paus. 10.4.4. Statues of Isis, Asclepius, and Sarapis, all standing side by side and made of marble were described by Pausanias in Aegira, Achaia (7.26.7). Marble statue in Epinoe: Paus. 2.29.1. Ivory in Cyllene, Elis: Str. 8.3.4. Gold and ivory in Sicyon: Paus. 2.10.3. Bronze in Gythium: Paus. 3.21.8; wood in Sparta: Paus. 3.14.7.

258 Paus. 2.30.1.

259 Paus. 2.27.2.

260 Anonymus, *De Incredibilibus*, 2.p. 89, 6–9.

261 πλεῖστα δέ σφισι καὶ θέας μάλιστα ἀγάλματα ἄξια τοῦ Ἀσκληπιοῦ παρέχεται τὸ ἱερόν. Paus. 4.31.10.

physician, Antonius Musa, 'through whose care he [sc. Augustus] had recovered from dangerous illnesses'.[262] These images were the work of some of the most renowned ancient artists. Both the work in Epidaurus and a beautiful bronze statue of Asclepius in Beroea were ascribed to the famous artist Phidias.[263] Alcamenes, a pupil of Phidias, was the creator of Asclepius' statue in Mantinea.[264] Strabo knew of a statue of Asclepius by Colotes in the village of Cyllene in Elis.[265]

Visuality was a particularly evocative factor in temples of Asclepius. Statues of the gods were prominent features in the architecture of the Pergamene Asclepieion. In fact, Petsalis-Diomidis argues that the architecture of the Pergamene Asclepieion, and an inscribed set of ritual rules which were provided for the convalescents, directed the movement and religious observances of the patients and formed the physical and conceptual context in which Aristides and his like experienced the process of healing.[266] An interpretation of the effect of the Asclepieion's space on Aristides' religious experience, and the ways in which this space was conditioned and constructed, involves an understanding of visuality in Aristides' day, as well as an intimate acquaintance with the *Lex Sacra*.[267] The sacred law itself was part of the patient's visual experience in the Asclepieion because it was publicly inscribed.

The inner space of the Asclepieion contained numerous visual testimonies of past patients expressing their gratitude to the god that healed them and reassured the present convalescents of the god's healing prowess. Indeed, viewers of works of art in Aristides' day were expected to look for implicit meanings within them.[268] The worshippers in the Asclepieion were inclined and even actively encouraged to read narratives of salvation into

---

262 *cuius opera ex ancipiti morbo convaluerat, statuam aere conlato iuxta signum Aesculapi statuerunt*. Suet. Aug. 59.

263 Epidaurus: Athenagoras, *Leg*. 17.4; Beroea: Lib. *Or*. 30.22–23.

264 Paus. 8.9.1.

265 Str. 8.3.4. This list is only a partial catalogue. For a collection of all the evidence see Edelstein & Edelstein vol. i (1945) T645–667.

266 Petsalis-Diomidis (2005) 185.

267 I use the term *Lex Sacra* to refer to an inscription which set out in detail the rules governing the ritual of incubation in the Asclepieion. The inscription was displayed at the entrance of the temple, welcoming and guiding the new patients. Another copy was also to be found in the courtyard. Petsalis-Diomidis (2005) 186, 199–203.

268 Cf. Achilles Tatius, *Leukippe and Kleitophon*, 1.2 (in the temple of Astarte), 3.6–8 (temple of Zeus of Mount Casius at Pelusium-paintings of Andromeda and Prometheus), 5.3–4 (painting of Prokne and Philomela; theory of interpreting a picture as a prophetic sign). Petsalis-Diomidis (2005) 207.

epigraphic votives—both textual and pictorial.[269] Local priests offered help to pilgrims in interpreting such enigmatic offerings of thanks.[270]

Statues, paintings and architecture enforced a cohesive visual language, and this visual language was universal. Coins, statues and other works of visual art portrayed similar patterns all over the Roman world.[271] They functioned as the teachers and educators of a common religious and ethical scheme.[272] Zanker has demonstrated the wide use of art objects, architecture and civic landscape as carriers of political, ethical and religious contents.[273] We see a similar unity of meanings and use of works of art in the religious sphere as well. Statues of the gods all over the οἰκουμένη displayed similar features.[274] The notion of visual theology is therefore seminal for appreciating the ritual evocations of Greek art as represented in the work of Aristides. It is also central to an examination of the religious dimension of images and the way these images affected Aristides' reception of Greek art. A comparison with other Second Sophistic authors confirms that Aristides was quite orthodox in this respect.[275]

Visual theology (that is, thinking about one's gods through their images) and visual culture, both resting on visual memory, account for much of Aristides' dream material. Statues of the gods appear regularly in Aristides' dreams.[276] In each of these instances Aristides understood these apparitions to be nightly visits of the gods themselves. Furthermore, Aristides' descriptions of the statues in his dreams were heavily influenced by the visual culture, as we learn, for example, from the following dream: 'at this point [in the dream] the god, in the posture in which he is represented in statues ...' (κἀν τούτῳ νεύει ἔξοδον ὁ θεὸς, ἔχων ἤδη τὸ ἑαυτοῦ σχῆμα ἐν ᾧπερ ἕστηκεν).[277] On another occasion Aristides had a daydream in which the 'Athena of Phidias in Athens' (σχῆμα οἵαπερ ἡ 'Αθήνησιν ἡ Φειδίου) appeared.[278]

---

[269] Petsalis-Diomidis (2005) 207.
[270] Cf. Plut. *De Pyth. Or.* 394e.
[271] Zanker (1988) 58.
[272] This function of visual culture is surprisingly overlooked in a recent and stimulating study of popular morality in classical antiquity by Morgan (2007).
[273] Zanker (1989) 46.
[274] Zanker (1989) 47, 58.
[275] Cf. Elsner (1996); for an anthropological study of ancient visions, dreams and function of images see: Clerc (1915) 9–85. A more general study of the history and theory of response to the power of images is that of Freedberg (1989).
[276] Cf. Aristid. *Or.* 47.10–14; 49.13; 47.17; 49.20; 49.21–22; 49.46 K.
[277] Aristid. *Or.* 50.50 K.
[278] Aristid. *Or.* 48.41 K.

The use of images in religious ritual accounts for their extensive presence in the imaginative and spiritual life of antiquity. The repetitive dressing, bathing and worship of images of the gods in festivals explains the vividness of Athena's image in Aristides' imagination, much as it accounts for Lucius' conception of Isis,[279] or Calasiris' mental image of Isis in Heliodorus' *Aethiopica*.[280] The visual language and the visual imagery of the Graeco-Roman world were responsible for much of its communication of religious messages. Aristides' divine knowledge and knowledge of the divine was shaped, to a large extent, by what he saw. Furthermore, due to the general tendency to convey contents via images and the capacity of works of visual art to act as semantic vehicles of communication there is no reason to assume that their impact on Aristides was exceptional. On the contrary, it is more plausible to assume that the impression these images left on Aristides and the particular manner in which visuality shaped his comprehension of the divine was similar to the impression these works of visual art left on the vast majority of their other spectators, particularly those of a similar cultural background.[281]

In the first part of this section I reviewed Aristides' behaviour from the point of view of pre-existing cultic habits. I considered the indoctrinating aspect of cult, festivals and games associated with Asclepius and demonstrated that they were highly effective cultural agents in the Graeco-Roman world. The second part then looked into the function of visual imagery as a vehicle of communication and the power of images to create visual theology. Specifically, I addressed the role of this visual culture in Aristides' religious experience. Tellingly, the apparitions of visual images of deities in Aristides' dreams and his identification of visual images with the gods themselves were shown to have echoed much wider cultural phenomena. It became evident that the role of visual culture and socially-organised cult had a profound effect on Aristides' religious life. Furthermore, I was able to demonstrate that this effect was very similar to the impact of these agents of culture on Aristides' contemporaries.

Therefore the conclusion that can be drawn from the two parts of this section concerns the profound effect of these agents of culture on the religious life of Aristides. In addition, I have shown that the impact of socially-

---

279 Apul. *Met.* 11.3–6, 24–25.

280 Heliod. *Aeth.* 7.8.7; Elsner (1996) 518.

281 That is, educated Greeks and Romans with a Greek education, predominantly but not exclusively male.

organised cult, of works of visual art, and of visual theology on Aristides was anything but exceptional. Rather than erroneously using the testimony of the *Sacred Tales* as evidence for the religious experience of a superstitious zealot, it is now possible to read the *Sacred Tales* as representative of much wider phenomena. The various components of Aristides' religious experience (such as convalescing in an Asclepieion, performing rites of cleansing, and incubation) reflected widespread and well-established forms of cult. Similarly, the recurrent appearances of images and statues of the gods in Aristides' dreams were to be expected in a world which laid such great emphasis on the representation of the gods and which relied so heavily on visual images as means of communication. Aristides' description of his reaction to visual imagery and cultic habits bears great resemblance to other testimonies from his age, notably the votive inscriptions from the Asclepieia and the work of Artemidorus. This role of visual culture and of social forms of cult-organisation within Graeco-Roman religious life reinforces the doubt cast upon the alleged dichotomy between 'private' and 'public' religions and the labelling of Aristides' religious experience as 'private' or 'personal'.

Conclusion

In the second chapter of this monograph I looked into society, disease and medicine in the *Sacred Tales*, asking how Aristides conceived of illness and what were the consequences of comprehending illness in this particular fashion. In the process, it became clear that medicine in Aristides' day and age was still anchored in other institutions, notably religion, and that Aristides' experience of being ill and seeking medical help was, to a large extent, religious. Furthermore, in the process of contextualizing the *Sacred Tales*, using corroborating pieces of evidence, I was able to demonstrate that the Graeco-Roman health-care system embraced a medical discourse which was unaware of a dichotomy between science and religion and between temple medicine and the scientific practice of medicine.

The third chapter concentrated on the religious aspect of the *Sacred Tales* by asking whether the religious experience of Aristides, as it is portrayed in his *Tales*, was representative of the Graeco-Roman world of the second half of the second century CE. I began by examining the theology of Aristides, with particular attention to his acquaintance with the myth of Asclepius. I then looked into some of the prevailing views and habits the classical world associated with divination through oracles and dreams because Aristides himself resorted to these religious institutions. I examined the educating power of cult and the visual environment on Aristides and compared its effect on him with other evidence about the indoctrinating faculty of visual culture in classical antiquity, using the works of modern scholarship.

Throughout the third chapter I was particularly interested in learning how influential the world around Aristides was in shaping his religious experience, and, viewed from the opposite perspective, how representative the religious experience Aristides recorded in his *Sacred Tales* was of his world. My findings were that none of the components of Aristides' religious experience was unique or even unorthodox. His theological frame of thought, his knowledge of Asclepius and his practice of divination represented common trains of thought in the Greek world during the high empire. The effect on Aristides of the visual environment (including both works of visual art and the role of public cult in temples, festivals and other religious ceremonies) bears great resemblance to the traces of the power of images and socially-organised cult in other sources. Finally, Aristides' narrative of his religious experience owed much to social institutions and to some of the most distinctive cultural phenomena in the Greek world of his age, which is often referred to as 'Second Sophistic'.[282] For Aristides, the bodily suffering was very much part of his religious experience. It is worth quoting Judith Perkins, who, reading Aristides in parallel with Ignatius of Antioch and with Marcus Aurelius, has concluded that 'if there is a pathology it belongs to the culture rather than to the psychology of any individual'.[283]

Having reviewed the mythology of Asclepius, the history of his cult and the theological conceptual scheme in which it was apprehended, it seems that the religious experience of Aristides was a 'product of its time' rather than a manifestation of eccentric behaviour and an unorthodox set of beliefs. Aristides' notion of the divine, its power and prowess, the ways of invoking the gods and the particular acts of grace each deity was likely to have granted resembled those which were taught by Greek tradition. While it is difficult to say for certain whether the religious life of Aristides was representative of his age, mainly because the *Sacred Tales* are unique in their subject matter and in their *raison d'être*, each component of this religious life can be seen as embodying its author's *Zeitgeist*.

---

282 These conclusions rest heavily on the first chapter.
283 Perkins (1995) 193.

CONCLUSION

This study has considered Aristides' portrayal of his experiences of falling ill and seeking medical help in their social, medical, and religious contexts. In particular I have focused on how Aristides envisaged his illness and the terms he used to understand and describe it. Initially I looked into the measures he took to address his medical condition. Particularly relevant here were the identities of those Aristides recognised as most suitable to offer health-care and the nature and origin of their authority. The seminal role of Asclepius and temple-healing in the medical history of Aristides, as well as the self-proclaimed nature of *Sacred Tales* as a work of eulogy to a benevolent god (who had saved Aristides from the grip of disease) raised some questions about the relations between temple medicine and scientific medicine in the world of the *Sacred Tales*; about the understanding of the discipline of medicine by a lay person; and about concepts of knowledge and belief in the world of Aristides.

Two general questions were always present. The first question was how representative a testimony Aristides' *Sacred Tales* are of the experiences of falling ill and seeking medical help in the Graeco-Roman world during the high empire. The second question was how reliable a testimony the *Sacred Tales* are of Aristides' experiences themselves. *Prima facie* the answers to both questions seemed to have been obvious. The *Sacred Tales* were not written by a physician or by an author who wished to compose a medical treatise. In fact, the *Sacred Tales* are rarely discussed by historians of ancient medicine. Most modern scholars who have read them dismiss the *Sacred Tales* as the testimony of a hypochondriac; a strange case of autobiography; the first among religious autobiographies or an epitome of an age of anxiety. It seemed unlikely, therefore, that such a work could offer a reliable and representative depiction of medical practices, of typical interactions between the sick and medical practitioners, as well as the general conceptual scheme in which ill-health was understood and which guided the sick in pursuit of health-care. Furthermore, the inclination of scholars to follow Philostratus and read the works of Aristides, particularly the *Sacred Tales*, as a work of a Second Sophistic implied that Aristides was consciously interested in glorifying himself as an author by the reworking of familiar themes.

However, existing scholarship on the *Tales* only offers a partial view. Aristides was seen as eccentric neither by his contemporaries nor by his late antique readers. He was a prominent member of the Greek world of Asia Minor, a distinguished man-of-letters and a personal acquaintance of at least one Roman emperor. Furthermore, no less an authority than Galen himself diagnosed Aristides as genuinely ill, and at the same time admired his strong character. This is not a depiction of a superstitious person or of a hypochondriac.

In order to examine this disparity between modern historians' views of Aristides and those of his contemporaries, it was necessary initially to consider the *Sacred Tales* themselves, including their method of composition and the motives behind them; their autobiographical character; and the comments of their ancient readers. Through this textual analysis it became possible to identify in the *Sacred Tales* a discernible narrative of redemption and a continuous thread of aretalogy. This critique therefore revealed that the *Sacred Tales* were an account of faith.

The second chapter then examined Aristides' portrayal of disease and medicine in their cultural and social contexts. Aristides' medical experiences occurred in a society which already had a recognisable medical discourse. I therefore analysed the grid of knowledge which regulated health-care activities in Aristides' world to examine how proficient Aristides was in using them; and to see to what extent his beliefs about disease and his therapeutic habits were derived from this grid.

In order to contextualise the experiences of Aristides within the appropriate social, medical and religious contexts I drew on the works of Kleinman and Geertz, among others, who argue that only after having learned how the various actors (such as the sick, the health-care providers, and the dream interpreters) in a particular social setting think and act about health-care, is it possible to evaluate the beliefs and actions of each individual. Moreover, conceptions of the nature of sickness and the measures taken to tackle it reveal the power structure which regulates medical discourse by denoting those people and texts which stood for medical authority.

The first section of the second chapter provided, therefore, a general overview of classical medicine. It demonstrated how Graeco-Roman health-care providers relied on various sources of medical authority. Some represented scholarly tradition; others could summon the help of the gods; while others relied on experience acquired over time. Although from the fifth century BCE medicine was seen as a discipline and as an art (both fell under the Greek term τέχνη), its foundations still overlapped with other spheres of knowledge, such as the philosophy of nature, cosmology and religion. Furthermore, Graeco-Roman medicine shared its vocabulary with these disciplines, which often led to some of its key notions having both a medical and a religious meaning. The use of similar notions in the fields of medicine and in other fields, notably religion, implied that the meaning of some of the most popular medical procedures could have equally belonged to scientifically-oriented medicine and to temple medicine. Likewise, the explanatory model used to understand illness could be traced back to the spheres of religion, cosmology, and philosophy of nature, as well as to scientific medicine. The seminal notion of 'cleansing' (κάθαρσις) was a case in point: cleansing had a medical meaning, applied in a situation where a physical imbalance had occurred (usually a collapse of the harmony between the four bodily fluids), and it often called for a physician to prescribe drugs (φάρμακα). 'Cleansing' (κάθαρσις) also had the religious meaning of negating defilement (μίασμα) and liquidating sin. The multiple meanings and uses of these notions left both the health-care providers who prescribed them, and those to whom they were being prescribed, free to decide what it connoted.

Another important theme which was considered was the nature of the relationship between Aristides the patient and his physicians. Ancient physicians were essentially craftsmen practising their trade. It was paramount for them to secure their patient's trust in order to guarantee their custom. As has been demonstrated, the most popular way for a physician to gain his clients' trust was by providing them with an accurate prognosis of the future course of their illness, which would exemplify the physician's professional skills. Such a display of his competence, in a world that did not have any institutionalised mechanism for guaranteeing that those professing to hold medical capabilities were actually up to the task, was the best way for a physician to persuade a prospective patient to put his faith in him. Aristides himself never used the term 'prognosis' although he did describe his physicians' perplexity and inability to recognise the nature of his disease. Furthermore, there were at least a few occasions when one might have expected a prognosis to have been provided (for example, in Rome in the early 140s, when Aristides arrived back in Smyrna from his unsuccessful journey to Rome, and when a growth appeared on his leg) and there is a general sense in the *Sacred Tales* of Aristides' that physicians' failed to secure his unqualified trust. It therefore seems that Aristides' reluctance to use the professional term 'prognosis' resulted from his physicians' inability to provide one. This was one of the reasons Aristides decided to turn to Asclepius.

As has been revealed, however, Aristides' choice of Asclepius was anything but eccentric. By the second century CE the cult of Asclepius was widespread all over the Graeco-Roman world and Asclepius was the most popular god of medicine. The Asclepieion in Pergamum had such an impressive reputation that it has been claimed Hadrian himself, as Roman emperor, remodelled it after his first imperial tour in the province of Asia.[1] Life in the Asclepieion offered Aristides frequent encounters with many of his social and intellectual peers, both Greek and Roman. The medical reputation of the temple was not disparaged even by the great Galen and, as we have seen, Aristides was able to consult some of the most distinguished physicians of his age while convalescing in the Asclepieion. According to the various votive offerings found in the Pergamene Asclepieion, as well as in many of the other Asclepieia, the convalescents used to spend a night of incubation during which the god might send them a dream with his prescription. In the morning the sick analysed the contents of their dreams with the help of their fellow worshippers and of the temple staff and followed the god's commands.

The *Sacred Tales* offer a record of over 130 dreams which Asclepius sent to Aristides. Most of these dreams were said to have contained medical advice. In the Graeco-Roman world dreams were commonly seen as autonomous entities rather than as a creation of the dreamer's mind. This view encouraged people to look and find god-sent messages within their dreams. Such an understanding of the nature of dreams, coupled with a firm belief in the gods and in their inclination to help mankind, explained the widespread phenomenon of dream-induced therapies in centres of religious healing throughout the Graeco-Roman world. Incubation was commonly practised in the various Asclepieia, as well as in temples of Sarapis and Isis. Divination in general and divination through dreams in particular was a central feature of Graeco-Roman religion. The physicians of the Graeco-Roman world, from Hippocrates through Herophilus and up until Galen, both acknowledged the existence of god-sent dreams and shared this common belief in divination. Perhaps more importantly, they all thought that dreams provided valuable information to the physician. Even Aristotle, who was of the minority view that divination through dreams was unfounded, acknowledged the widespread nature of this belief and supported the use of dreams for medical care. Equally revealing was the comparison of Aristides' understanding of dreams with that of his contemporary dream-interpreter, Artemidorus of Daldis. Interpretation of dreams was common in the Graeco-Roman world and many of the themes which come up in the work of Artemidorus and

---

[1] There is, however, insufficient evidence to argue conclusively that Hadrian himself, as emperor, refurbished the Pergamene Asclepieion, cf. Le Glay (1976); Petsalis-Diomidis (2010) 167, 184, 193.

other professional dream-interpreters have a close resemblance to those found in the *Sacred Tales*. Together with the realisation that Artemidorus' approach to dreams and dream-interpretation shared common elements with that of one of the major medical schools of classical antiquity (the empiricist school), it became clear that Aristides' approach to dreams, his acceptance of their divine origin, and his keenness to follow the divine messages he identified within them, mark him representative of his age.

In the first section of chapter two I was able to demonstrate that the Graeco-Roman health-care system, by which I referred to the conceptual scheme which guided all health-related activities in the Graeco-Roman world, never forced the sick to choose between a religious and a scientific explanatory model of disease. The most popular beliefs about illness included scientific elements, in the form of mechanistic explanations of cause and effect, but also left room for cosmological, philosophical, and religious explanations. The meaning of some of the commonest prescriptions Aristides received, such as cleansing and the use of drugs, explained why he never had to choose between the explanatory model offered by his physicians and that of temple medicine. Graeco-Roman health-care never regarded the two as mutually exclusive.

The vivid description of the sick, medicine, and of physicians which emerged from the *Sacred Tales* in the second section of chapter two, elucidated many of the general traits of Graeco-Roman health-care, as seen from the patient's point of view. Aristides' testimony indicates that the sick were active members of society, rather than being banished to its margins. The patients in the Pergamene Asclepieion, according to the *Sacred Tales*, participated in the vibrant civic life of Pergamum and the Asclepieion itself attracted intellectuals and members of the Graeco-Roman elite from far and wide. In addition, the *Sacred Tales* clearly recognised a discernible group of health-care providers, who were marked by the title 'physician' (ἰατρός). Another important group of health-care providers in Aristides' record were the priests in the Pergamene Asclepieion. These two groups, however, were not mutually exclusive. On the contrary, according to the *Sacred Tales*, they shared a common professional language, prescribed similar treatments, and were like-minded in their approach to dreams and to their place in medical treatment. Perhaps even more telling was Aristides' depiction of one of the two temple-wardens as a physician and temple warden interchangeably.

Medical praxis, according to the *Sacred Tales*, included in addition to the general rule of following Asclepius' commands, the letting of blood, horseback riding, walking barefooted and cleansing. According to the votive offerings of grateful worshippers Asclepius offered identical prescriptions to many of his other patients. Dream-induced therapy, however, is the single most important medical procedure that Aristides underwent. It appears, though, that all medical authorities—both physicians and priests—shared Aristides' conviction that these dreams were god-sent and that it would be wise to follow them to the letter. Furthermore, in many instances Aristides consulted physicians and priests about the accurate interpretation of these dreams and their true meaning. On the evidence of the *Sacred Tales*, there was no challenge to this understanding of the dream-mechanism by any health-care provider.

In the third section of chapter two I endeavoured to write a medical history of Aristides in which his pathologies, the way he envisaged them and his dialectic relationship with the prevailing health-care authorities would be addressed. One of the most noticeable features of Aristides' medical history, as it emerged from the *Sacred Tales*, was that he made no attempt to understand what was clinically wrong with him. Unlike his later admirer, the Greek rhetor Sopater, who diagnosed Aristides as epileptic, Aristides himself never provided a diagnosis of his illness. Furthermore, when encountering health-care providers, be they physicians, priests, or Asclepius, Aristides showed no interest in a clinical diagnosis. Likewise, he never evaluated any of the treatment-options offered to him in term of cause and effect. The probable reason for this omission is that Aristides did not envisage illness or health-care in terms which encouraged or allowed for such a sequence. A second pre-eminent theme in Aristides' medical history was his oratorical career and how his recuperation and professional success were inherently connected.

The symbiotic connection between professional success and the teleological character of the *Sacred Tales* themselves led to an inquiry into the religious aspect of the medical experiences Aristides wrote up in the *Sacred Tales*. Throughout the *Sacred Tales* Aristides attributed a deep religious meaning to his illness, and he depicted his recuperation as salvation. In the third chapter I looked into the religious aspects of Aristides' medical experiences—namely looking at religion as a cultural system; contextualizing the experiences of Aristides within this cultural system; and finally asking how representative were Aristides' beliefs and cultic habits of the prevailing religious climate of his day—using the same critical tools as those used in the second chapter and asking similar questions, such as how representative was Aristides' religious experience.

The general question behind the inquiry of the third chapter revolved around the definition of Aristides' religious experience as a 'personal' or 'private' religion by some modern scholars, and the reading of the *Sacred*

Tales as an epitome of an age of anxiety. In the first section I was able to recount Aristides' knowledge of theology and relate it to the teachings of Greek *paideia*. I demonstrated that his views about the Greek pantheon, the nature of the gods, the genealogy of the different gods and their mutual hierarchy, reflected Greek tradition. In the second section I looked into Aristides' portrayal of Asclepius. Aristides was a devout worshipper of Asclepius and it was important to demonstrate that his acquaintance with the myth of Asclepius; the expectations Aristides had of this particular deity; and the cultic habits he practised echoed the vast majority of ancient sources. Furthermore, in light of the popularity of the cult of Asclepius in the second century CE, not only among Greeks but among Romans as well, Aristides' decision to approach Asclepius when ill was typical of Graeco-Roman behaviour.

The next section examined the means Aristides used to invoke the gods. As mentioned above, perhaps the most compelling argument for describing the religious experience of Aristides as personal or private is the abundance of occurrences where he communicated directly with a god. However, having examined Aristides' understanding of divination, oracles, and god-sent dreams it became evident that Aristides relied on a wide range of institutions to teach him how to use these religious phenomena, as well as to instruct him about their very existence and nature. This investigation emphasised how misleading a title 'personal' or 'private' religion is for Aristides' religious experience.

Finally, in section four, I considered the formative role of society in moulding Aristides' religious beliefs and habits into their particular shape by looking at the function of visual culture and social forms of cult-organisation. Aristides was a keen participant in religious cult, festivals, and games. These events functioned as some of the most effective *loci* for creating communal identity and for transmitting religious ideas. Hymns, images, and patterns of cult conveyed religious meanings and taught those who were present about the nature of the various gods, retold their myths, and recalled past acts of grace the gods had bestowed upon their worshippers. Equally evocative were works of visual art, which were shown to have functioned as semantic vehicles of communication. Particularly heuristic was a comparison of the impact of visual culture on Aristides with its effect on other Second Sophistic authors and on the dream interpreter, Artemidorus. These comparisons proved that Aristides and other sophists saw similar content in works of visual art. Moreover, the comparison with the *Oneirokritika* of Artemidorus has shown that Aristides understood the apparitions of images of gods in his dreams in the accustomed manner of Graeco-Roman dream-interpreters. Both these comparisons, as well as the general survey of the power of images in classical antiquity, provided sufficient evidence to substantiate the claim that the religious experience of Aelius Aristides was a product of his time, and that the *Sacred Tales* captured some of the most seminal traits of Graeco-Roman culture of the second half of the second century CE.

Aristides embodied in his writing the fears and beliefs that were characteristic of his age. His written work belongs to the category of the Second Sophistic; the fears caused by his illness were a sensitive seismograph of a wider attention to the fragility of the human body, particularly in the years which followed the great plague of 165 CE; Aristides' belief in the power of Asclepius to heal him, alongside his appeal to other types of health-care providers, notably physicians, represented typical choices of a sick individual in the Graeco-Roman world. However, Aristides' picture of his life and times is unique in its perspective. The focus of the *Sacred Tales* was his own experiences, fears, and beliefs. Unlike the works of historians, the *Sacred Tales* were not an endeavour to present a general picture of the Roman Empire. Unlike some other authors, such as Plutarch and Tertullian, Marcus Aurelius and Ignatius of Antioch, the *Sacred Tales* were not offering a general commentary on contemporary religious life. Unlike Philostratus' *Lives of the Sophists*, the *Sacred Tales* showed no interest in the general contribution of the sophist to his city. Rather, the *Sacred Tales* revolve solely around Aristides' own experiences. In consequence, they offer a rare view of the particular ways in which general patterns of politics, religion, and health manifested themselves in an élite individual's experience.

BIBLIOGRAPHY

Abu Ali, A. (1992): *The Medical Writings of Rufus of Ephesus* (Ph.D thesis: University of London).

Allan, N. (2001): 'The physician in ancient Israel', *Medical History* 45: 377–394.

Aleshire, S.B. (1989): *The Athenian Asclepieion* (Amsterdam).

Amundsen, D.W. (1996): *Medicine, Society and Faith in the Ancient and Mediaeval Worlds* (Baltimore).

Anderson, G. (1986): *Philostratus* (London).

———. (1989): 'The *Pepaideumenos* in action: Sophists and their outlook in the early empire', *ANRW* ii. 33. 1: 79–208.

———. (1993): *The Second Sophistic: A Cultural Phenomenon in the Roman Empire* (London).

Andersson, P. and Roos, B.B. (1997): 'On the psychology of Aelius Aristides', *Eranos* 95: 26–38.

Andrei, O. (1984): *A. Claudius Charax di Pergamo: Interessi Antiquari e Antichità Cittadine nell'età degli Antonini* (Bologna).

Artelt, W. (1937): *Studien zur Geschichte der Begriffe "heilmittel" und "gift": Urzeit, Homer, Corpus Hippocraticum* (Leipzig).

Auffarth, C. (2004): 'Festivals', *DNP* 5: 396–406.

Avotins, I. (1971): Review of Behr 1968, *AJPh* 92: 347–349.

Baal, J.V. (1971): *Symbols for Communication* (Assen).

Bakhtin, M. (1981): *The Dialogic Imagination: Four Essays* (Austin).

Bal, M. (1985): *Narratology: Introduction to the Theory of Narrative* (Toronto).

Baldwin, B. (1992): 'The career and works of Scribonius Largus', *Rh. Mus.* 135: 74–82.

Banton, M. (ed. 1966): *Anthropological Approaches to the Study of Religion* (London).

Barasch, M. (1992): *Icon: Studies in the History of an Idea* (New York and London).

Barnes, J. (1991): 'Galen on logic and therapy', in Kudlien and Durling 1991: 50–102.

Barnes, J. and Jouanna, J. (eds. 2003): *Galien et la Philosophie* (Genève).

Barthes, R. (1977): 'Introduction to the structural analysis of narratives', in R. Barthes *Image, Music, Text* (New York), 79–124.

Barton, T.S. (1994): *Power and Knowledge: Astrology, Physiognomics, and Medicine Under the Roman Empire* (Ann Arbor).

Baslez, M.-F., Hoffmann, P. and Pernot, L. (eds. 1993): *L'Invention de l'Autobiographie d'Hésiode à Saint Augustine: Actes du Deuxième Colloque de l'Equipe de Recherche sur l'Hellénisme post-Classique* (Paris).

Bates, D. (ed. 1995): *Knowledge and the Scholarly Medical Traditions* (Cambridge).

Baumgarten, R. (1998): *Heiliges Wort und heilige Schrift bei den Griechen: hieroi logoi und verwandte Erscheinungen* (Tübingen).

Beard, M., North, J. and Price, S. (1998): *Religions of Rome* (Cambridge).

Beard, M. (1986): 'Cicero and divination: the foundation of a Latin discourse', *JRS* 76: 33–46.

Behr, C. (1968): *Aelius Aristides and the Sacred Tales* (Amsterdam).
———. (1981–1986) (trans.): *P. Aelius Aristides: The Complete Works* i–ii (Leiden).
———. (1994): 'Studies on the biography of Aelius Aristides', *ANRW* ii. 34.2: 1140–223.
Bianchi, U. (1973): 'The history of religions and the "religio-anthropological approach"', in L. Honko, (ed.) *Science of Religion* (The Hague), 299–321.
Birley, A.R. (1987): *Marcus Aurelius* 2nd edn. (London).
———. (1997): *Hadrian: the Restless Emperor* (London).
———. (2000): 'Hadrian to the Antonines', *CAH* XI²: 132–194.
Björck, G. (1946): '"Οναρ ἰδεῖν: De la perception de la rêve chez les anciens', *Eranos* 44: 306–314.
Bompaire, J. (1989): 'La sacré dans les discours d'Aelius Aristide', *REG* 102: 28–39.
———. (1993): 'Quatre styles d'autobiographie au II siècle après J.-C.: Aelius Aristide, Lucien, Marc-Aurèle, Galien', in Baslez, Hoffmann, and Pernot 1993: 199–209.
Bouché-Leclercq, A. (1879): *Histoire de la Divination dans l'Antiquité* (Paris).
Boudon, V. (1994): 'Le rôle de l'eau dans les prescriptions médicales d'Asclépios chez Galien et Aelius Aristide', in Ginouvès, Guimier-Sorbets, Jouanna, and Villardeds 1994: 157–168.
Boulanger, A. (1923): *Aelius Aristide* (Paris).
Boulogne, J. (1996): 'Plutarque et la médicine', *ANRW* ii. 37.2: 2762–2792.
Bowersock, G. (1969): *Greek Sophists in the Roman Empire* (Oxford).
———. (1994): *Fiction as History* (Berkeley).
Bowie, E.L. (1970): 'Greeks and their past in the Second Sophistic', *P&P* 46: 3–41.
———. (1982): 'The importance of sophists', *YCS* 27: 29–60.
———. (2000): 'Literature and sophistic', *CAH* XI²: 898–921.
———. (2006): 'Choral performances', in D. Konstan and S. Said, (eds.) *Greeks on Greekness, Supplement to the Proceedings of the Cambridge Philological Society* (Cambridge), 69–92.
Bowra, C.M. (1968): *Pindar* (Oxford).
Brock, J. (1929): *Greek Medicine* (London).
Brock, R. (2000): 'Sickness in the body politic: medical imagery in the Greek polis', in V.M. Hope and R. Marshall, (eds.) *Death and Disease in the Ancient City* (London), 24–34.
Brunt, P.A. (1994): 'The bubble of the Second Sophistic', *BICS* 39: 25–52.
Buraselis, K. (2000): 'Kos. Between Hellenism and Rome: Studies on the Political, Institutional and Social History of Kos from ca. the Middle Second Century BC until Late Antiquity', *TAPS* 90, Part 4.
Burford, A. (1969): *The Greek Temple Builders at Epidauros: A Social and Economic Study of Building in the Asklepian Sanctuary, During the Fourth and Early Third Centuries B.C.* (Liverpool).
Burkert, W. (1972): *Lore and Science in Ancient Pythagoreanism* (Cambridge).
———. (1985): *Greek Religion* (Cambridge).
———. (1992): *The Orientalizing Revolution: Near Eastern influence on Greek Culture* (Cambridge).

Cameron, A. (2004): *Greek Mythography in the Roman World* (Oxford).
Cavallero, M. (1975–1976): 'Un liberto 'prega' per Augusto e per le gentes: *CIL* VI 30975', *Helikon* 15–16: 146–186.
Champeaux, L.J. (1990a): 'Sors Oraculis: les oracles en Italie sous le République et l'Empire', *MÉFRA* 102: 271–302.
——. (1990b): '"Sorts" et divination inspirée. Pour un préhistoire des Italiques', *MÉFRA* 102: 801–828.
Chaniotis, A. (1995): 'Illness and cures in the Greek propitiatory inscriptions and dedications of Lydia and Phrygia', in Van der Eijk, Horstmanhoff, and Schrijvers 1995: 323–344.
Clerc, C. (1915): *Les Théories Relatives au Culte des Images chez les Auteurs Grecs du IIme Siècle Après J. C.* (Paris).
Cohan, S. and Shires, L.M. (1988): *Telling Stories: A Theoretical Analysis of Narrative Fiction* (London).
Cohn-Haft, L. (1956): *The Public Physicians of Ancient Greece* (Northampton).
Cortés Copete, J.M. (1999): *Discursos. 5* (Madrid).
Cox Miller, P. (1994): *Dreams in Late Antiquity: Studies in the Imagination of a Culture* (Princeton).
Craik, E. (2010): 'The Teaching of Surgery', in: H.F.J. Horstmanshoff (ed.): *Hippocrates and Medical Education* (Leiden).
Croon, J.H. (1967): 'Hot Springs and healing Gods', *Mnemosyne* 40: 225–246.
Cuddon, J.A. (1991): *A Dictionary of Literary Terms and Literary Theory* (Oxford).
Cuomo, S. (2007): *Technology and Culture in Greek and Roman Antiquity* (Cambridge).
Currie, B. (2005): *Pindar and the Cult of Heroes* (Oxford).
Deichgräber, K. (1965): *Die griechische Empirikerschule, Sammlung der Fragmente und Darstellung der Lehre* (Berlin).
——. (1970): *Medicus gratiosus: Untersuchungen zu einem griechischen Artzbild: Mit dem Anhang Testamentum Hippocratis und Rhazes' De indulgentia medici* (Wiesbaden).
Derrida, J. (1981): *Dissemination* (Oxford).
Desanti, L. (1990): *Sileat omnibus perpetuo divinandi curiositas: Indovini e Sanzioni nel Diritto Romano* (Milano).
Deubner, L. (1900): *De Incubatione* (Leipzig).
——. (1932): *Attische Feste* (Berlin).
Deuse, W. (1993): 'Celsus im Prooemium von "De Medicina": Römische Aneignung griechischer Wissenschaft', *ANRW* ii. 37.1: 819–841.
Dillon, J. (1977): *The Middle Platonists* (London).
Dodds, E.R. (1951): *The Greeks and the Irrational* (Berkeley).
——. (1965): *Pagan and Christian in an Age of Anxiety* (Cambridge).
——. (1973): 'The ancient idea of progress', in E.R. Dodds *The Ancient Concept of Progress and Other Essays on Greek Literature and Belief* (Oxford) 1–26.
LiDonnici, L.R. (1995): *The Epidaurian Miracle Inscriptions* (Atlanta).
Douglas, M. (1966): *Purity and Danger* (London).
Downie, J. (2008): 'Proper pleasures: bathing and oratory in Aelius Aristides' *Hieros Logos I* and *Oration 33*', in Harris and Holmes 2008: 115–130.
Duncan-Jones, R.P. (1996): 'The impact of the Antonine plague', *JRA* 9: 108–136.

Edelstein, L. (1937): 'Greek medicine in its relation to religion and magic', *Bulletin of the Institute of the History of Medicine* 5: 201–246.
Edelstein, E. and Edelstein, L. (1998): *Asclepius*, vols. i–ii (Baltimore) (first published 1945).
Edelstein, L. (1967): *Ancient Medicine* (Baltimore).
Van der Eijk, Ph.J. (1995): 'Aristotle on 'distinguished physicians' and on the medical significance of dreams', in Van der Eijk, Horstmanhoff, and Schrijvers 1995: 447–459.
Van der Eijk, Ph., Horstmanhoff, H.F.J. and Schrijvers, P.H. (eds. 1995): *Ancient Medicine in its Socio-Cultural Context* vols. i–ii. (Amsterdam).
Elsner, J. (1991): 'Cult and sculpture: sacrifice in the Ara Pacis Augustae', *JRS* 81: 50–61.
———. (1992): 'Pausanias: a Greek pilgrim in the Roman world', *P&P* 135: 3–29.
———. (1996): 'Image and ritual: reflections on the religious appreciation of classical art', *CQ* 46: 515–531.
———. (2007) 'Physiognomics: Art and text', in S. Swain, (ed.) *Seeing the Face, Seeing the Soul: Polemon's Physiognomy from Classical Antiquity to Medieval Islam*, (Oxford), 203–224
Evans-Pritchard, E.E. (1965): *Theories of Primitive Religion* (Oxford).
Ferguson, J. (1970): *The Religions of the Roman Empire* (London).
Festugière, A.J. (1945): *La Révélation d'Hermès Trismégiste. Vol. 1 L'Astrologie et les Sciences Occultes: avec un Appendice sur l'Hermétisme Arabe* (Paris).
———. (1954): *Personal Religion Among the Greeks* (Berkeley).
———. (1967): 'Lettre du médicin Thessalos à Claude ou Néron', *Hermétisme et mystique païnne* (Paris), 155–163.
———. (1986): *Aelius Aristide, Discours Sacrés: Rêve, Religion, Médecine au IIe Siècle Après J.-C.* (Paris).
Firth, R. (1973): *Symbols Public and Private* (Cornell).
Fisher, S. and Greenberg, R.P. (1977): *The Scientific Credibility of Freud's Theories and Therapy* (Hassocks and New York).
Flacelière R. (1976): *Greek Oracles* (London).
Flinterman, J.J. (1995): *Power, Paideia and Pythagoreanism* (Amsterdam).
Foucault, M. (1989): *The Archaeology of Knowledge* (London).
———. (1989): *The Birth of the Clinic* (London).
Fowler, R.L. (2000): *Early Greek Mythography* (Oxford).
Fraser, P.M. (1960): 'Two studies on the cult of Sarapis in the Hellenistic world', *Opuscula Atheniensia* 3:1–54.
Frazer, J.G. (1900): *The Golden Bough* (London).
Frede, M. (1981): 'On Galen's epistemology', in Nutton 1981: 65–86.
———. (1982): 'The method of the so-called Methodical school of medicine', in J. Barnes, J. Brunschwig, M. Burnyeat and M. Schofield, (eds.) *Science and Speculation* (Cambridge), 1–23.
———. (2003): 'Galen's theology', in Barnes and Jouanna 2003: 73–126.
Freedberg, D. (1989) *The Power of Images* (Chicago).
Freud, S. (1991): *The Interpretations of Dreams* (London: edited by J. Strachey).
Furley, M.D. and Bremer, J.M. (2001): *Greek Hymns* vol. i–ii (Tübingen).
Gamberale, L. (1987): 'Il voto del sacerdote *C. Manius Felix Fortunatianus*: una

dedica poetica a Saturno Africano', in *Filologia Forme letterarie: Studi Offerti a Francesco Della Corte*, 5 vols. (Urbino), vol. iv: 397–417.
Gay, P. (1985): *Freud for Historians* (Oxford).
Geertz, C. (1973): *The Interpretation of Cultures* (New York).
Genette, G. (1980): *Narrative Discourse* (Oxford).
Gilliam, J.F. (1961): 'The plague under Marcus Aurelius', *AJPh* 82: 225–251.
Ginouvès, R., Guimier-Sorbets, A.-M., Jouanna, J. and Villardeds, L. (eds. 1994): *L'Eau, la Santé et la Maladie dans le Monde Grec* (Paris).
Le Glay, M. (1976): 'Hadrien et l'Asklépieion de Pergame', *BCH* 100: 347–372.
Good, B.J. (1994): *Medicine, Rationality and Experience: An Anthropological Perspective* (Cambridge).
Goody, J. (1977): *The Domestication of the Savage Mind* (Cambridge).
Gorrini, M.E. (2005): 'The Hippocratic impact on healing cults: the archaeological evidence in Attica', in: P. van der Eijk (ed.) *Hippocrates in Context* (Leiden) 133–156.
Gourevitch, D. (1984): *Le Triangle Hippocratique dans le Monde Gréco-Romain: le Malade, sa Maladie et son Médecin* BEFAR 251 (Rome).
———. (1991): 'Le pratique méthodique', in P. Mudry and J. Pigeaud, (eds.) *Les Écoles Médicales à Rome* (Geneva), 51–81.
Gourevitch, M. and Gourevitch, D. (1968): 'Le cas Aelius Aristide ou mémoires d'un hystérique au IIe siècle', *Informations Psychiatriques* 14: 897–902.
Graf, F. (1992): 'Heiligtum und Ritual: das Beispiel der griechisch-römischen Asklepieia', in S. Albert, (ed.) *Le Sanctuaire Grec* (Genève), 159–203.
Grant, M. (2000): *Galen on Food and Diet* (London).
Grant, R.L. (1960): 'Antyllus and his medical works', *Bulletin of the History of Medicine* 34: 154–174.
Griffiths, J.G. (1975): *Isis in the Metamorphoses of Apuleius* (Groningen).
Grmek, M.D. (1989): *Diseases in the Ancient World* (Baltimore).
———. (ed. 1998): *Western Medical Thought from Antiquity to the Middle Ages* (Cambridge).
Grodzynski, D. (1974): 'Superstitio', *REA* 76: 36–60.
Guarducci, M. (1978): *Epigrafia Greca, IV: Epigrafi Sacre Pagane e Cristiane* (Rome).
Guey, J. (1948): 'Encore la "pluie miraculeuse"', *RP* 22: 16–62.
Guillon, J. (1983): 'Essai de diagnostic médical (somatique) de la maladie d'Aelius Aristide', *Littérature, Médicine et Société* 5: 83–90.
Habicht, C. (1969): *Die Inschriften des Asklepieions* (Berlin).
Hahn, J. (1991): 'Plinius und die griechischen Ärzte in Rom: Naturkonzeption und Medizinkritik in der Naturalis Historia', *Sudhoffs Archiv* 75: 209–239.
Halbwachs, M. (1992): *On Collective Memory* (Chicago).
Halfmann, H. (1979): *Die Senatoren aus dem östlichen Teil des Imperium Romanum: bis zum Ende des 2. Jahrhunderts n. Chr.* (Göttingen).
Hamilton, J.S. (1989): 'Scribonius Largus and the medical profession', *Bulletin of the History of Medicine* 60: 209–216.
Hankinson, R.J. (1992): 'Doing without hypotheses: the nature of *Ancient Medicine*', in J.A. Lopez Ferez, (ed.) *Tratados Hipocráticos: (Estudios Acerca de su Contenido, Forma y Influencia): Actas del VIIe Colloque International Hippocratique* (Madrid), 55–68.

———. (1989): 'Galen and the best of all possible worlds', *CQ* 39: 206–227.
———. (1992): 'Galen's philosophical eclecticism', *ANRW* ii. 36.5: 3505–3522.
———. (1998a): *Causes and Explanation in Ancient Greek Thought* (Oxford).
———. (ed. 1998b): *Galen: On Antecedent Causes* (Cambridge).
———. (ed. 2007): 'The man and his work', in R.J. Hankinson (2007) *The Cambridge Companion to Galen* (Cambridge) 1–33.
Hanson, A.E. and Green, M.H. (1996): 'Methodicorum princeps; Soranus of Ephesus', *ANRW* ii.37.2: 1834–1855.
Hanson, J.S. (1980): 'Dreams and vision in the Graeco-Roman world and early Christianity', *ANRW* ii. 23.2: 1395–427.
Harris, W.V. (1989): *Ancient Literacy* (Cambridge).
———. (2003): 'Roman opinions about the truthfulness of dreams', *JRS* 93: 18–34.
Harris, W.V. and Holmes, B. (eds. 2008): *Aelius Aristides Between Greece and Rome* (Leiden).
Harrison, S. (1996): 'Apuleius' *Metamorphoses*', in G.L. Schmeling, (ed.) *The Novel in the Ancient World* [*Mnemosyne Suppl. 159*] (Leiden), 491–516.
Harrison, S.J. (2000–2001): 'Apuleius, Aelius Aristides and religious autobiography', *Anc. Narr.* 1: 245–259.
Harrison, T. (2007): *Greek Religion* (London).
Hazard-Guillon, C. (1983): 'La névrose d'Aelius Aristide. Étude de la psychologie morbide d'Aelius Aristide dans les Discours sacrés', *LMS* 5: 91–114.
Helman, C. (1984): *Culture, Health and Illness* (Bristol).
Henrichs, A. (2003): '"Hieroi Logoi" and "Hierai Bibloi": the (un)written margins of the sacred in ancient Greece', *HSCP* 101: 207–266.
Hoffmann, A. (1998): 'The Roman remodelling of the Asclepieion', in H. Koester, (ed.) *Pergamon, Citadel of the Gods* (Harrisburg Pa.).
Holmes, B. (2008): 'Aelius Aristides' illegible body', in Harris and Holmes 2008:81–114.
Hölscher, T. (2004): *The Language of Images in Roman Art* (Cambridge).
Hornblower, S. (1994): 'Narratology and narrative techniques in Thucydides', in S. Hornblower, (ed.) *Greek Historiography* (Oxford), 131–166.
Horrocks, C. and Jevtic, Z. (1997): *Introducing Foucault* (New York).
Horstmanshoff, H.F.J. (1990): 'The ancient physician: craftsman or scientist?', *Journal of the History of Medicine and Allied Sciences* 45: 176–197.
———. (2004) "'Did the god learn medicine?' Asclepius and Temple Medicine in Aelius Aristides' Sacred Tales", *Magic and Rationality in Ancient Near Eastern and Graeco-Roman Medicine*, Horstmanshoff, H.F.J. & Stol, M. (eds.), Leiden/Boston: Brill, pp. 325–342.
Isaac, B. (2004): *The Invention of Racism in Classical Antiquity* (Princeton).
Israelowich, I. (2007): 'The world of Aelius Aristides', *SCI* 26: 92–110.
———. (2008): 'The rain miracle of Marcus Aurelius: (Re-) construction of consensus', *G&R* 55(1): 83–102.
Jackson, R. (1988): *Doctors and Diseases in the Roman Empire* (London).
———. (1990): 'Waters and spas in the classical world', in R. Porter, (ed.) *The Medical History of Waters and Spas: Medical History* [*Suppl.*] 10: 1–13.
———. (1992): 'Spas, waters and hydrotherapy in the Roman world', in J. DeLaine and D.E. Johnston, (eds.) *Roman Baths and Bathing: Journal of Roman Archaeology* [*Suppl. Series*] 37: 107–116.

Jackson, S.W. (1969): 'Galen on mental disorders', *Journal of the History of Behavioural Science* 5: 365–384.

Jaeger, W. (1957): 'Aristotle's use of medicine as model of method in his ethics', *JHS* 77: 54–61.

James, W. (1982): *The Varieties of Religious Experience* (London).

Jameson, M.H. (1986): 'Sophocles, Antigone 1005–1022. An illusion', in M. Cropp, E. Fantham, and S.E. Scully, (eds.) *Greek Tragedy and its Legacy: Studies Presented to D.J. Conacher* (Calgary), 59–66.

———. (1991): 'Sacrifice before battle', in V.D. Hanson, (ed.) *Hoplites: the Classical Greek Battle Experience* (London), 197–227.

Johnston, I. (2006): *Galen on Disease and Symptoms* (Cambridge).

Jones, C.P. (1991): 'Aelius Aristides On the Water in Pergamon', *Archäologischer Anzeiger* 1991: 111–117.

———. (1998): 'Aelius Aristides and the Asclepieion', in H. Koester, (ed.) *Pergamon, Citadel of the Gods* (Harrisburg Pa.) 63–78.

De Jong, I.J.F. and Sullivan, J.P. (eds. 1994): *Modern Critical Theory and Classical Literature* (Leiden).

Jordanova, L. (1995): 'The social construction of medical knowledge', *Social History of Medicine* 8(3): 361–381.

Jost, M. (1985): 'Sanctuaires et cultes d'Arcadie', *Étud. Pélop.* 9: 202–210.

Jouanna, J. (1978): 'Le médecin modèle du législateur dans les Lois de Platon', *Ktèma* 3: 77–91.

———. (1980a): 'Médecine et politique dans la Politique d'Aristote (II 1268b25–1269a28)', *Ktèma* 5: 257–266.

———. (1980b): 'Politique et médecine. La problématique du changement dans le Régime des maladies aiguës et chez Thucydide (livre vi)' in M.D. Grmek, (ed.) *Hippocratica. Actes du Colloque Hippocratique de Paris* (Paris), 299–319.

———. (1998): 'L'interprétation des rêves et la théorie micro-macro cosmique dans la traité hippocratique *Du Régime*: sémiotique et mimesis', in K.D. Fisher, D. Nickel, and P. Potter, (eds.) *Text and Tradition* (Leiden), 161–174.

———. (1999): *Hippocrates* (Baltimore).

———. (2003a): *La Maladie Sacrée* (Paris).

———. (2003b): 'La notion de nature chez Galien', in Barnes and Jouanna 2003: 229–262.

Kallet, L. (1999); 'The diseased body politic, Athenian public finance, and the massacre at Mykalessos (Thucydides 7.27–29)', *AJPh* 120 (2): 223–244.

Kessels, A.H.M. (1969): 'Ancient systems of dream-classification', *Mnemosyne* 22: 389–424.

Klein, R. (1981): *Die Romrede des Aelius Aristides: Einführung* (Darmstadt).

———. (1983): *Die Romrede des Aelius Aristides* (Darmstadt).

Kleinman, A. (1980): *Patients and Healers in the Context of Culture* (Berkeley).

Knibbe, D. (1981–1982): 'Neue Inschriften aus Ephesos VIII', *JÖAI* 53: 87–150.

Kollesch, J. (1981): 'Galen und die Zweite Sophistik', in Nutton 1981: 1–11.

Kripke, S. (1982): *Wittgenstein: On Rules and Private Language* (Oxford).

Krug, A. (1985): *Heilkunst und Heilkult: Medizin in der Antike* (Munich).

Kudlien, F. (1981): 'Galen's religious belief', in Nutton, 1981: 117–130.

Kudlien, F. and Durling, R.J. (eds. 1991): *Galen's Methods of Healing* (Leiden).
Kuhn, T. (1962): *The Structure of Scientific Revolutions* (Chicago).
La Barre, W. (1972): *The Ghost Dance* (New York).
Lane Fox, R. (1986): *Pagans and Christians* (London).
Lang, M. (1977): *Cure and Cult in Ancient Corinth* (Connecticut).
Langslow, D.R. (1994): 'Celsus and the makings of Latin medical terminology', in G. Sabbah and P. Mudry, (eds.) *La Médecine de Celse: Aspects Historiques, Scientifiques et Littéraires* 13: 297–318.
———. (1999): 'The language of poetry and the language of science: the Latin poets and medical Latin', in J.N. Adams and R.G. Mayer, (eds.) *Aspects of the Language of Latin Poetry: Proceedings of the British Academy* 93: 183–226.
Laskaris, J. (2002): *The Art is Long: On the Sacred Disease and the Scientific Tradition* (Leiden).
Lejeune, P. (1975): *Le Pacte Autobiographique* (Paris).
Lenz, F.W. (1959): *The Aristides Prolegomena* (Leyden).
Leven, K.-H. (1993): 'Miasma und Metadosis—antike Vorstellungen von Ansteckung', *Medizin, Gesellschaft und Geschichte* 11: 44–73.
Lévi-Strauss, C. (1966): *The Savage Mind* (London).
Liebeschuetz, J.H.W.G. (2000): 'Religion', *CAH* XI^2: 987–1008.
Littman R.J. and Littman, M.L. (1973): 'Galen and the Antonine plague', *AJPh* 94: 243–255.
Lloyd, G.E.R. (1979): *Magic, Reason, and Experience* (Cambridge).
———. (1982): *Science, Folklore and Ideology* (Cambridge).
———. (1991): *Methods and Problems in Greek Science* (Cambridge).
———. (2003): *In the Grip of Disease* (Oxford).
Lloyd-Jones, H. (1983): *The Justice of Zeus* (Berkeley).
Lonie, I.M. (1981): *The Hippocratic Treatises "On Generations", "On the Nature of the Child", "Diseases IV": A Commentary* (Berlin).
Lonnoy, M.G. (1986): 'L'expérience initiatique d'Aelius Aristide', *BAGB*: 41–50.
MacMullen, R. (1976): *Roman Government's Response to Crisis, A.D. 235–337* (New Haven).
———. (1981): *Paganism in the Roman Empire* (New Haven).
Magie, D. (1950): *Roman Rule in Asia Minor* (Princeton).
Mannhardt, T.W.E. (1904): *Wald und Feldkulte* (Berlin).
Marwood, M. (1984): 'A reappraisal of the altar of Iulius Apolinaris at Corbridge, Northumberland', *Latomus* 43: 316–335.
Mason, H.J. (1974): *Greek Terms for Roman Institutions: A Lexicon and Analysis* (Toronto).
Mattern, S.P. (2008): *Galen and the Rhetoric of Healing* (Baltimore).
Mattes, J. (1970): *Der Wahnsinn im griechischen Mythos und in der Dichtung bis zum Drama des V.Jh.* (Heidelberg).
Merlin, A. (1944): *Inscriptions Latines de la Tunisie* (Paris).
Michenaud, G. and Dierkens, J. (1972): *Les Rêves dans les "Discours Sacrés" d'Aelius Aristide, IIe Siècle ap. J.-C. Essai d'Analyse Psychologique Publié à l'Initiative et avec le Concours de Roland Crahay* (Mons).
Millar, F. (1977): *The Emperor in the Roman World (31 B.C.-A.D. 337)* (London).
Misch, G. (1950): *A History of Autobiography in Antiquity* (London).

Momigliano, A. (1966): *Studies in Historiography* (New York).
Morgan, T. (2007): *Popular Morality in the Early Empire* (Cambridge).
Motschmann, C. (2002): *Die Religionspolitik Marc Aurels* (Stuttgart).
Moulinier, L. (1952): *Le Pur et l'Impur dans la Pensée des Grecs d'Homère à Aristote*, Etudes et Commentaires 12 (Paris).
Mudry, P. (1982): *La Préface du De medicina de Celse: Texte, Traduction et Commentaire* (Rome).
Müller, H. (1987): 'Ein Heilungsbericht aus dem Asklepieion von Pergamon', *Chiron* 17: 193–233
Nicosia, S. (1984): *Elio Aristide: Discorsi Sacri* (Milan).
Nijhuis, K. (1995): 'Greek doctors and Roman patients', in Van der Eijk, Horstmanhoff, and Schrijvers 1995: 49–67.
Nilsson, M.P. (1906): *Griechische Feste von religiöser Bedeutung: mit Ausschluss der attischen* (Leipzig).
Nisbet, R. and Hubbard, M. (1970): *A Commentary on Horace's Odes: Book 1* (Oxford).
Nock, A.D. (1933): *Conversion* (Oxford).
Norman, A.F. (1953): 'Philostratus and Libanius', *CP* 48: 20–23.
North, J. (1990): 'Diviners and divination at Rome', in: M. Beard and J. North, (eds.) *Pagan Priests* (Cornell), 49–71.
Nutton, V. (1971a): 'Two notes on immunities: Digest 27, 1, 6, 10 and 11', *JRS* 61: 53–62.
———. (1971b): 'L. Gellius Maximus, physician and procurator', *CQ* 21: 262–272.
———. (ed. 1981): *Galen: Problems and Prospects* (London).
———. (1996): 'Antyllus', *DNP* 1: 817–818.
———. (2000): 'Medicine', *CAH* XI^2: 943–965.
———. (2001): 'Satyrus', *DNP* 11: 125.
———. (2004): *Ancient Medicine* (London).
Oberhelman, S.M. (1991): *The Oneirocriticon of Achmet: a Medieval Greek and Arabic Treatise on the Interpretation of Dreams* (Texas).
———. (1993): 'Dreams in Graeco-Roman medicine', *ANRW* ii. 37.1: 121–156.
Oliver, J.H. (1953): *The Ruling Power* (Philadelphia).
Pack, R. (1947): 'Two sophists and two emperors', *CP* 42: 17–20.
Padel, R. (1992): *In and Out of the Mind: Greek Images of the Tragic Self* (Princeton).
Palm, J. (1959): *Rom, Römertum und Imperium in der griechischen Literatur der Kaiserzeit* (Lund).
Palmer, R.E.A. (1976): 'Jupiter blaze, gods of the hills, and the Roman topography of *CIL* VI 377', *AJA* 80: 43–56.
Palmer, R. (1990): *Studies of the Northern Campus Martius in Ancient Rome* (TAPhS 80.2, Philadelphia).
Parker, R. (1983): *Miasma* (Oxford).
———. (1996): *Athenian Religion* (Oxford).
Pearcy, L.T. (1988): 'Theme, dream and narrative: reading the Sacred Tales of Aelius Aristides', *TAPA* 118: 377–391.
Pease, A.S. (1920–1923): *Cicero De Divinatione* (Illinois).
Pelling, C. (1997): 'Tragical dreamer: some dreams in the Roman historians', *G&R* 44: 197–213.
Penso, G. (1984): *La Médecine Romaine: l'Art d'Esculape dans la Rome Antique* (Paris).

Perkins, J. (1995): *The Suffering Self: Pain and Narrative Representation in the Early Christian Era* (London).
Pernot, L. (1997): *Éloges Grecs de Rome* (Paris).
Petit, C. (2010): 'Hippocrates in the pseudo-Galenic Introduction: Or how was medicine taught in Roman times?' in: Manfred (H.F.J.) Horstmanshoff (ed.). Hippocrates and Medical Education (Leiden),
Petsalis-Diomidis, A. (2005): 'The body in space: visual dynamics in Graeco-Roman healing pilgrimage', in J. Elsner and I. Rutherford, (eds.) *Seeing the Gods: Pilgrimage in Graeco-Roman & Early Christian Antiquity* (Oxford), 183–218.
———. (2006a): 'Sacred writing, sacred reading: the function of Aelius Aristides' self-presentation as author in the Sacred Tales', in B. McGing, and J. Mossman, (eds.) *The Limits of Ancient Biography* (Swansea), 193–212.
———. (2006b): 'Amphiaraos present: images of healing pilgramege in ancient Greece', in R. Shepard and R. Maniura (eds.) *Images and Presence: Esseays on the Presence of the Prototype within the Images* (Ashgate), 205–229.
———. (2008): 'The body in the landscape: Aristides' *corpus* in the light of the *Sacred Tales*', in Harris and Holmes 2008: 131–150.
———. (2010): *Truly Beyond Wonders* (Oxford).
Phillips, E.D. (1952): 'A hypochondriac and his god', *G&R* 61: 23–36.
Pleket, H. (1995): 'The social status of physicians in the Graeco-Roman world', in Van der Eijk, Horstmanshoff and Schrijvers 1995: 27–34.
Polito, R. (1999): 'On the life of Asclepiades of Bithynia', *JHS* 119: 48–66.
Poole, F.J.P. (1986): 'Metaphors and maps: towards comparison in the anthropology of religion', *Journal of the American Academy of Religion* 3: 411–457.
Porter, D. (1995): 'The mission of social history of medicine: An historical view', *Social History of Medicine* 8(3): 345–359.
Porter, R. (1985): 'The patient's view: doing medical history from below', *Theory and Society* 14: 175–198.
———. (1987): *Disease, Medicine and Society in England 1550–1860* (London).
———. (1998): *The Greatest Benefit to Mankind: A Medical History of Humanity from Antiquity to the Present* (New York).
Price, S. (1984): *Rituals and Power: The Roman Imperial Cult in Asia Minor* (Cambridge).
———. (1999): *Religions of the Ancient Greeks* (Cambridge).
———. (2004): 'The future of dreams: from Freud to Artemidorus', in R. Osborne, (ed.): *Studies in Ancient Greek and Roman Society* (Cambridge), 226–259.
Prince, G. (1987): *A Dictionary of Narratology* (London).
Pritchett, W.K. (1979): *The Greek State at War 3* (London).
Puech, B. (2002): *Orateurs et Sophistes Grecs dans les Inscriptions d'Époque Impériale* (Paris).
Purcell, N. (1996): 'Pliny the Elder', *OCD* 3rd edn.
Quet, M.H. (1993): 'Parler de soi pour louer son dieu: le cas d'Aelius Aristide', in Baslez, Hoffmann, and Pernot 1993: 211–251.
Radt, W. (1988): *Pergamon: Geschichte und Bauten, Funde und Erforschung einer antiken Metropole* (Cologne).
Rawson, E. (1982): 'The life and death of Asclepiades of Bithynia', *CQ* 32: 358–370.
Reardon, B.P. (1971): *Courants Littéraires Grecs des IIe et IIIe Siècles après J.-C'* (Paris).

——. (1993): 'L'autobiographie à l'époque de la Seconde Sophistique: quelques conclusions', in Baslez, Hoffmann, and Pernot 1993: 279–284.
Renberg, G. (2003): *Commanded by the Gods: An Epigraphical Study of Dreams and Visions in Greek and Roman Religious Life* (Ph.D thesis: Duke University).
Ricoeur, P. (1984): *Time and Narrative* (Chicago).
Rivkin, J. and Ryan, M. (2004): *Literary Theory: an Anthology* (Oxford).
Robert, L. (1969): 'Lioracle de Claros', in Ch. Delvoye and G. Roux, (eds) *La Civilation Grecque de l'Antiquité à nos Jours* (Brussels), 305–312.
Roesch, P. (1982): 'Le culte d'Asklépios à Rome', in: G. Sabbach (ed.) *Médecins et mécine dans l'antiquité* (Paris), 171–179.
——. (1985): 'Le sanctuaire d'A. Alipheira en Arcadie', *BSABR* 3: 22–32.
Rubensohn, O. (1902): 'Paros III. Das Asklepieion', *MDAI(A)* 27: 199–238.
Rubinstein, G. (1985): *The Methodist Method* (Ph.D. thesis: Cambridge University).
Russell, D.A. (1973): *Plutarch* (London).
——. (1992): *Dio Chrysostom: Orations VII, XII, XXXVI* (Cambridge).
Russell, D.A. and Wilson, N.G. (1981): *Menander Rhetor* (Oxford).
Rutherford, I. (1999): 'To the land of Zeus ... patterns of pilgrimage in Aelius Aristides', *Aevuum Antiquum* 12:133–148.
——. (2001): *Pindar's Paeans: A Reading of the Fragments With a Survey of the Genre* (Oxford).
Samama, E. (2003): Les Médecins dans le Monde Grec: Sources Épigraphiques sur la Naissance d'un Corps Médical (Genève).
Sandbach, F. (1975): *The Stoics* (New York).
Schäfer, P. (1997): *Judeophobia: Attitudes Toward the Jews in the Ancient World* (Cambridge, Mass.).
Scheid, J. (1985): 'Religion et superstition à l'époque de Tacite. Quelques réflexions', in *Religión, Superstición y Magía en el Mundo Romano* (Cádiz), 19–34.
Schmid, W. (1887–1897): *Der Atticismus in seinen Hauptvertretern: von Dionysius von Halikarnass bis auf den zweiten Philostratus* (Stuttgart).
Schmitz, T. (1997): *Bildung und Macht: zur sozialen und politischen Funktion der zweiten Sophistik in der griechischen Welt der Kaiserzeit* (Munich).
——. (2006): *Modern Literary Theory and Ancient Texts: An Introduction* (Oxford).
Schofield, M. (1986): 'Cicero for and against divination', *JRS* 76: 47–65.
Schröder, H.O. (1986): *Publius Aelius Aristides: Heilige Berichte* (Heidelberg).
Sheppard, A.R.R. (1984): 'Homonoia in the Greek cities of the Roman Empire', *Anc. Soc.* 15: 229–252.
Sherwin-White, S. (1978): *Ancient Cos* (Göttingen).
Singer, P.N. (1997): *Galen: Selected Works* (Oxford).
Skorupski, J. (1976): *Symbol and Theory* (Cambridge).
Smith, N.D. (1989): 'Diviners and divination in Aristophanic comedy', *Cl. Ant.* 5: 140–158.
Sokolowski, F. (1973): 'On the New Pergamene *Lex Sacra*', *GRBS* 14: 407–413.
Spawforth, A.J. and Walker, S. (1985): 'The world of the Panhellenion. I. Athens and Eleusis', *JRS* 75: 78–104.
Spiro, M.E. (1973): 'Symbolism and functionalism in the anthropological study of religion', in L. Honko, (ed.) *Science of Religion* (The Hague), 322–339.

Von Staden, H. (1989): *Herophilus* (Cambridge).
Sternberg, M. (1977): *Expositional Modes and Temporal Ordering in Fiction* (Baltimore).
Stone, L. (1981): *The Past and the Present* (Boston and London).
Van Straten, F.T. (1976): 'Daikrates' dream. A votive relief from Kos, and some other kat'onar dedications', *BABesch* 6: 1–38.
———. (1981) 'Gifts of the gods', in: H.S. Versnel (ed.): *Faith Hope and Worship* (Leiden), 65–151.
———. (1988): 'The god's portion in Greek sacrificial representations. Is the tail doing nicely?', in R. Hägg, (ed.) *Early Greek Cult Practice* (Stockholm), 51–68.
Swain, S. (1996): *Hellenism and Empire* (Oxford).
———. (2004): 'Sophists and emperors: the case of Libanius', in S. Swain and M. Edwards, (eds.) *Approaching Late Antiquity: The Transformation from Early to Late Empire* (Oxford), 355–400.
———. (ed. 2007): *Seeing the Face, Seeing the Soul: Polemon's Physiognomy from Classical Antiquity to Medieval Islam* (Oxford).
Syme, R. (1939): *The Roman Revolution* (Oxford).
Temkin, O. (1971): *The Falling Sickness*, 2nd ed. (Baltimore).
———. (1977): *The Double Face of Janus* (Baltimore).
———. (1991): *Hippocrates in the World of Pagans and Christians* (Baltimore).
Tomlinson, R.A. (1983): *Epidauros* (London).
Trapp, M. (2007): 'Philosophy, scholarship, and the world of learning', in J. Elsner, S. Harrison, and S. Swain, (eds.) *Severan Culture* (Cambridge), 470–488.
Turcan, R. (1996): *The Cults of the Roman Empire* (Oxford).
Véligianni, C. (1994): 'Lex sacra aus Amphipolis', *ZPE* 100: 391.
Veyne, P. (1976): *Le Pain et le Cirque: Sociologie Historique d'un Pluralisme Politique* (Paris).
———. (1987): 'De Halai en Dalmatie. Un vœu de voyageur et les rêves chez Virgile', *Poikilia: Études Offertes à Jean-Pierre Vernant* (Paris), 381–395.
Walde, C. (1999): 'Dream interpretation in a prosperous age? Artemidorus, the Greek interpreter of dreams', in Shulman, D. and Stroumsa, G.G., (eds.) *Dream Cultures. Explorations in the Comparative History of Dreaming* (New York and London).
———. (2004): 'Dreams; Interpretation of dreams', *DNP* 4: 714–719.
Wallace, A.F.C. (1966): *Religion: An Anthropological View* (New York).
Wallace-Hadrill, A. (1983): *Suetonius: The Scholar and his Caesars* (London).
Weber, M. (1968): *On Charisma and Institution Building* (ed.) S.N. Eisenstadt (Chicago).
Weinreich, O. (1914): 'Typisches und Individuelles in der Religiosität des Aelius Aristides', *Neue Jahrbücher für das classische Altertum, Geschichte und deutsche Literatur* 33: 597–602.
Weiss, C. (1998): *Literary Turns: The Representation of Conversion in Aelius Aristides' Hieroi Logoi and Apuleius' Metamorphoses* (Ph.D thesis: University of Yale).
West, M. (1983): *The Orphic Poems* (Oxford).
White, H. (1980): 'The value of narrativity in the representation of reality', *Critical Inquiry* 7: 5–27.
———. (1984): 'The question of narrative in contemporary historical theory', *History and Theory* 23: 1–33.

———. (1987): *The Content of Form* (Baltimore).
Whitehorne, J.E.G. (1977): 'Was Marcus Aurelius a hypochondriac?', *Latomus* 36: 413–421.
Whitmarsh, T. (2001): *Greek Literature and the Roman Empire: the Politics of Imitation* (Oxford).
———. (2006): *The Second Sophistic* (Cambridge).
Wilamowitz-Möllendorf, U. von (1925): 'Der Rhetor Aristides', *SB. Berl. Akad.* 28: 333–358.
Winkler, J.J. (1985): *Auctor and Actor: A Narratological Reading of Apuleius' Golden Ass* (Berkeley).
Wissowa, G. (1912): *Religion und Kultus der Römer* 2nd edn. (Munich).
Wittgenstein, L. (1968): *Philosophical Investigations* (Oxford).
Wöhlers, M. (1999): *Heilige Krankheit: Epilepsie in antiker Medizin, Astrologie und Religion* (Marburg).
Woodman, A.J. (1977): *Velleius Paterculus: The Tiberian Narrative, 2.94–13* (Cambridge).
Woolf, G. (1994): 'Becoming Roman, staying Greek', *PCPhS* 40: 116–143.
Wörrle, M. (1969): 'Die Lex sacra von der Hallenstrasse (Inv. 1965, 20)' in Habicht 1969: 167–190.
Zanker, P. (1988): *The Power of Images in the Age of Augustus* (Ann Arbor).

INDEX

www.ingramcontent.com/pod-product-compliance
Ingram Content Group UK Ltd.
Pitfield, Milton Keynes, MK11 3LW, UK
UKHW020846290926
15470UKWH00004B/1586

9 789004 229082